ORTHOPEDIC CLINICS OF NORTH AMERICA

www.orthopedic.theclinics.com

Sports-Related Injuries

October 2020 • Volume 51 • Number 4

ELSEVIER

1600 John F. Kennedy Boulevard • Suite 1800 • Philadelphia, Pennsylvania, 19103-2899.

http://www.orthopedic.theclinics.com

ORTHOPEDIC CLINICS OF NORTH AMERICA Volume 51, Number 4
October 2020 ISSN 0030-5898, ISBN-13: 978-0-323-79599-9

Editor: Lauren Boyle
Developmental Editor: Kristen Helm

Orthopedic Clinics of North America (ISSN 0030-5898) is published quarterly by Elsevier Inc., 360 Park Avenue South, New York, NY 10010-1710. Months of issue are January, April, July, and October. Business and Editorial Offices: 1600 John F. Kennedy Blvd., Suite 1800, Philadelphia, PA 19103-2899. Customer Service Office: 3251 Riverport Lane, Maryland Heights, MO 63043. Periodicals postage paid at New York, NY and additional mailing offices. Subscription prices are $344.00 per year for (US individuals), $786.00 per year for (US institutions), $403.00 per year (Canadian individuals), $960.00 per year (Canadian institutions), $471.00 per year (international individuals), $960.00 per year (international institutions), $100.00 per year (US students), $100.00 per year for (Canadian students), $220.00 per year for (international students). Foreign air speed delivery is included in all *Clinics* subscription prices. All prices are subject to change without notice. **POSTMASTER:** Send change of address to *Orthopedic Clinics of North America,* **Elsevier Health Sciences Division, Subscription Customer Service, 3251 Riverport Lane, Maryland Heights, MO 63043. Customer Service (orders, claims, online, change of address): Elsevier Health Sciences Division, Subscription Customer Service, 3251 Riverport Lane, Maryland Heights, MO 63043. Tel: 1-800-654-2452 (U.S. and Canada); 314-447-8871 (outside U.S. and Canada). Fax: 314-447-8029. E-mail:** journalscustomerservice-usa@elsevier.com **(for print support);** journalsonlinesupport-usa@elsevier.com **(for online support).**

Reprints. For copies of 100 or more, of articles in this publication, please contact the Commercial Reprints Department, Elsevier Inc., 360 Park Avenue South, New York, NY 10010-1710. Tel.: 212-633-3874; Fax: 212-633-3820; E-mail: reprints@elsevier.com.

Orthopedic Clinics of North America is covered in MEDLINE/PubMed (Index Medicus), Cinahl, Excerpta Medica, and Cumulative Index to Nursing and Allied Health Literature.

EDITORIAL BOARD

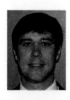

CONTRIBUTORS

AUTHORS

JOHN D. (JD) ADAMS Jr. MD
Assistant Professor, Department of
Orthopedic Surgery, Division of Orthopedic
Trauma, Prisma Health, Greenville Memorial
Medical Hospital, Greenville, South Carolina,
USA

CHRISTOPHER S. AHMAD, MD
Professor and Chief of Sports Medicine,
Department of Orthopedic Surgery, Columbia
University Irving Medical Center, New York,
New York, USA

SYED S. AHMED, MBChB, LLM, MSc, FRCS
(Tr & Orth)
University College London Hospital NHS
Foundation Trust, London, United Kingdom

FORREST L. ANDERSON, MD
Resident Physician, Department of
Orthopedic Surgery, Columbia University
Irving Medical Center, New York, New York,
USA

FREDERICK M. AZAR, MD
Department of Orthopaedic Surgery and
Biomedical Engineering, University of
Tennessee-Campbell Clinic, Memphis,
Tennessee, USA

TYLER J. BROLIN, MD
Department of Orthopaedic Surgery and
Biomedical Engineering, University of
Tennessee-Campbell Clinic, Memphis,
Tennessee, USA

JAMES H. CALANDRUCCIO, MD
Associate Professor, Department of
Orthopaedic Surgery and Biomechanical
Engineering, University of Tennessee-
Campbell Clinic, Memphis, Tennessee, USA

ALLISON E. CREPEAU, MD
Division of Sports Medicine, UConn Health,
Farmington, Connecticut, USA; Orthopaedic
Surgeon, Elite Sports Medicine at

Connecticut Children's, Hartford,
Connecticut, USA

WISSAM S. FAWAZ, MD
Clinical Fellow, Department of Orthopaedic
Surgery, University of British Columbia,
Vancouver, British Columbia, Canada

NATHAN L. GRIMM, MD
Orthopaedic Surgeon, Team Physician, Boise
State University, Idaho Sports Medicine
Institute, Boise, Idaho, USA; Division of Sports
Medicine, UConn Health, Farmington,
Connecticut, USA

FARES S. HADDAD, BSc, MD (Res),
MCh(Orth), FRCS(Orth), FFSEM
University College London Hospital NHS
Foundation Trust, The Institute of Sports,
Exercise and Health, The Princess Grace
Hospital, London, United Kingdom

ANDREW E. JIMENEZ, MD
Orthopaedic Surgeon, UConn Health, Division
of Sports Medicine, Farmington, Connecticut,
USA

DEREK KELLY, MD
Professor, Department of Orthopaedic
Surgery and Biomechanical Engineering,
University of Tennessee-Campbell Clinic,
Memphis, Tennessee, USA

BRIAN J. KISTLER, MD
Assistant Professor, Department of
Orthopedic Surgery, SUNY Upstate Medical
University, Syracuse, New York, USA

MICHAEL L. KNUDSEN, MD
Assistant Professor, Department of
Orthopedic Surgery, University of Minnesota,
Minneapolis, Minnesota, USA

SUJITH KONAN, MBBS, MD (Res), MRCS,
FRCS(Tr &Orth)
University College London Hospital NHS
Foundation Trust, London, United Kingdom

JAMES LEE PACE, MD
Orthopaedic Surgeon, Elite Sports
Medicine at Connecticut Children's, Hartford,
Connecticut, USA; Division of Sports
Medicine, UConn Health, Assistant Professor,
Department of Orthopedics, Farmington,
Connecticut, USA; Team Physician,
Quinnipiac University, Hamden, Connecticut,
USA

BENJAMIN J. LEVY, MD
Orthopaedic Surgeon, Division of Sports
Medicine, UConn Health, Farmington,
Connecticut, USA

MARKUS F. LOEFFLER, MD, MA
Orthopedic Resident, Department of
Orthopedic Surgery, Prisma Health, Greenville
Memorial Medical Hospital, Greenville, South
Carolina, USA

AHMED A. MAGAN, BM, BSc, MRCS,
FRCS(Tr & Orth)
University College London Hospital
NHS Foundation Trust, London, United
Kingdom

BASSAM A. MASRI, MD, FRCSC
Professor and Head, Department of
Orthopaedic Surgery, University of British
Columbia, Vancouver, British Columbia,
Canada

BENJAMIN MAUCK, MD
Assistant Professor, Department of
Orthopaedic Surgery and Biomechanical
Engineering, University of Tennessee-
Campbell Clinic, Memphis, Tennessee, USA

MARTIN J. O'MALLEY
Hospital for Special Surgery, New York, New
York, USA

DAVID PARKER, MD
University of Tennessee-Campbell
Clinic Orthopedis, Memphis, Tennessee,
USA

JAVAD PARVIZI, MD, FRCS
Director of Clinical Research, The Rothman
Institute, Thomas Jefferson University,
Philadelphia, Pennsylvania, USA

KARAN A. PATEL
Mayo Clinic, Phoenix, Arizona, USA

BRUCE PATON, BAppSc, PhD
University College London Hospital NHS
Foundation Trust, The Institute of Sports,
Exercise and Health, London,
United Kingdom

SIERRA G. PHILLIPS, MD
Department of Orthopaedic Surgery and
Biomechanical Engineering, University of
Tennessee-Campbell Clinic, Memphis,
Tennessee, USA

CHARLES A. POPKIN, MD
Associate Professor, Department of
Orthopedic Surgery, Columbia University
Irving Medical Center, New York, New York,
USA

IAN POWER, MD
Orthopedic Associates P.A., Farmington, New
Mexico, USA

ANNA RAMBO, MD
Foot and Ankle Fellow, Department of
Orthopaedic Surgery and Biomechanical
Engineering, University of Tennessee-
Campbell Clinic, Memphis, Tennessee,
USA

DAVID J. RUTA, MD
Bellin Health Titletown Sports Medicine and
Orthopedics, Green Bay, Wisconsin, USA

BENJAMIN SHEFFER, MD
Assistant Professor, Department of
Orthopaedic Surgery and Biomechanical
Engineering, University of Tennessee-
Campbell Clinic, Memphis, Tennessee, USA

RICHARD A. SMITH, PhD
Department of Orthopaedic Surgery and
Biomedical Engineering, University of
Tennessee-Campbell Clinic, Memphis,
Tennessee, USA

ZACHARY L. TELGHEDER, MD
Department of Orthopedic Surgery, SUNY
Upstate Medical University, Syracuse, New
York, USA

NORFLEET B. THOMPSON, MD
Department of Orthopaedic Surgery and
Biomechanical Engineering, University of
Tennessee-Campbell Clinic, Memphis,
Tennessee, USA

THOMAS W. THROCKMORTON, MD
Department of Orthopaedic Surgery and
Biomedical Engineering, University of
Tennessee-Campbell Clinic, Memphis,
Tennessee, USA

WILLIAM J. WELLER, MD
Department of Orthopaedic Surgery and
Biomechanical Engineering, University of

Tennessee-Campbell Clinic, Memphis,
Tennessee, USA

STEVEN YACOVELLI, BS
Clinical Research Fellow, The
Rothman Institute, Thomas Jefferson
University, Philadelphia, Pennsylvania,
USA

CONTENTS

Femoroacetabular impingement results from a mismatch of congruency between the femoral head and the acetabulum. This condition is most common among young, active patients and may lead to pain, decreased quality of life, and inability to participate in athletics. Hip preservation surgery is widely performed is used as a definitive treatment option in athletes at all levels of competition. Athletes have reported high rates of return to play and satisfaction and expect rehabilitation to require approximately 4 to 6 months. This article provides an overview of femoroacetabular impingement, including diagnosis and treatment, with focus on athletes and return to play.

It is essential for total knee arthroplasty patients to return to their previous level of activity to maintain a healthy lifestyle. This article reviews the current recommendations regarding return to physical activity after total knee arthroplasty and trying to find the balance between levels of activity and prosthetic joint preservation. In general, most total joint replacement patients are able to return to their previous level of activity and to a lesser extent to sports. This article discuss patients' actual levels of activity including their return to work and sport and the factors that influence meeting their expectations for surgery.

Psychosocial health may influence the outcomes after total knee arthroplasty (TKA). We investigated the hypothesis that multimodal therapy influences the quality of life and function in patients diagnosed with osteoarthritis of the knee joint. Secondly, in patients who then proceed to have TKA post-multimodal therapy, does the response to the multimodal therapy influence the overall functional outcome of surgery? Patients diagnosed with osteoarthritis of the knee were enrolled in the study and prospectively followed-up. A total of 526 patients were enrolled and available for the study. All participants were enrolled for 12 classes of 60-minute duration over 6-weeks. Apart from an exercise program, the class also included physiotherapist-led education and a 'weight management' lecture by a dietitian. In summary, the multimodal therapy program improved the SF-12, OKS, pain scores (visual analogue scale) and WOMAC scores significantly. The multimodal therapy protocol can optimize patients' psychological scores prior to TKA and may enhance ultimate functional outcome.

SPORTS-RELATED INJURIES

PREFACE

Each year in the United States, over 3.5 million pediatric athletes and approximately 2 million high-school athletes suffer sports-related injuries. Professional athletes suffer more than 2000 injuries per 10,000 participants, placing them among the top 5 most-injured occupations. It's no surprise, then, that a large percentage of orthopedic patients are athletes. Whether amateurs or professionals, most athletes are highly motivated to recover and rehabilitate and get back in the game. The articles in this issue provide practical pointers and valuable information about the treatment of orthopedic sports-related injuries, from hand fractures to hip impingement.

Femoroacetabular impingement has been studied extensively in the past several years, with numerous authors noting the difficulty of diagnosis and treatment of this condition. Parvizi and Yacovelli describe the multifaceted path to diagnosis and treatment, in addition to the rehabilitation protocol after hip preservation surgery in athletes, noting that 82% return to sport. Although total joint arthroplasty generally is not associated with athletic injuries, indications are expanding to younger and more active patients and, as noted by Masri and Fawaz, patients' expectations from total joint replacement surpass pain control and quality of life to include sports and athletic activities. Masri and Fawaz identify factors that influence patients' achievement of their expectations. Observing that psychosocial health plays an important role in patients with osteoarthritis who have total joint arthroplasty, Magan and coauthors describe a multimodal therapy protocol that improves patient-reported outcomes after operative or nonoperative treatment in both physical and mental scores after primary total knee arthroplasty.

Musculoskeletal injuries are frequent in skiing and snowboarding, sports in which participation continues to increase. Injuries may involve the upper or lower extremities or the spine. Kistler and Telgheder note that recognition of risk factors and injury patterns can aid in the diagnosis and treatment of these often complex orthopedic injuries. They describe the unique injuries related to their environment, pathomechanics, and equipment. Adams and Loeffler focus on the complex bony and soft tissue injuries that accompany tibial plateau fractures and require comprehensive evaluation and meticulous planning. They provide a description of the general approach considerations in the treatment of these injuries.

Sports-related injuries are frequent in children and adolescents, and Grimm and colleagues and Mauck and colleagues provide valuable information on patellar injuries and distal radial physeal injuries. For these conditions, correct diagnosis is paramount to developing a surgical plan that will yield the most favorable outcome for these young athletes. Grimm and colleagues discuss treatment options ranging from minimally invasive all-arthroscopic treatment to open ligament reconstruction, tibial tubercle osteotomy, and trochleoplasty for patellar instability. Mauck and colleagues describe the radiographic criteria for the diagnosis of stress injuries of the distal radial physis and discuss conservative and operative treatment.

Overuse wrist injuries are a common problem in athletes and can be related to tendinopathies or osteoarticular pathologic condition. Phillips describes possible results of overuse, including tendinopathies and osteoarticular issues, such as impaction syndromes, impingement syndromes, and stress injuries, as well as their conservative treatment and operative treatment for refractory cases. Weller and colleagues discuss the treatment of scaphoid fractures, the most frequent carpal fracture in athletes. The radiographic criterion for operative is described, and percutaneous and open techniques are discussed.

As athletes begin sports specialization at increasingly earlier ages, evidence is growing that early sports specialization is associated with increased injury risk in general, but especially in throwing athletes. Anderson and colleagues describe how parents and coaches strongly influence the young athlete's choice to specialize early, often to the athlete's detriment. They make a strong case for diversification in sports participation for the physical and psychological well-being of these developing athletes. Shoulder injuries are frequent in throwing athletes, and severe enough involvement can require shoulder arthroplasty. Power and colleagues identify factors associated with an increase in major complications with the use of indwelling interscalene nerve catheters and suggest that patients with pulmonary comorbidities

Orthop Clin N Am 51 (2020) xv–xvi
https://doi.org/10.1016/j.ocl.2020.07.002
0030-5898/20/© 2020 Published by Elsevier Inc.

may benefit from alternative pain management strategies to avoid complications in the early postoperative period.

The management of Achilles tendon rupture continues to be controversial in the everyday athlete; however, O'Malley and Patel review the evidence that in elite athletes, surgical intervention generally is preferred. They describe their operative technique and postoperative protocol in the management of Achilles tendon injuries in elite athletes. Ruta and Parker emphasize that Jones fractures in both elite and recreational athletes are best treated with surgical fixation, given superior results as compared with nonoperative management. They give pointers for operative fixation and discuss return-to-play guidelines.

The authors in this issue have provided information on the diagnosis and treatment of a number of sports-related injuries in both recreational and elite athletes. We hope readers will find this information valuable in their treatment of these injuries.

Frederick M. Azar, MD
Department of Orthopaedic Surgery
University of Tennessee–Campbell Clinic
1211 Union Avenue, Suite 510
Memphis, TN 38104, USA

E-mail address:
fazar@campbellclinic.com

Knee and Hip Reconstruction

Return to Sports After Joint Preservation Hip Surgery

Steven Yacovelli, BS, Javad Parvizi, MD, FRCS*

KEYWORDS

- Femoroacetabular impingement • Hip preservation • Athlete • Return to sport

KEY POINTS

- Diagnosis of femoroacetabular impingement (FAI) is multifaceted. Careful consideration of clinical presentation, physical examination, and diagnostic imaging is necessary to reach the correct diagnosis.
- Rehabilitation protocol for the athlete consists of 3 main phases: (1) partial weight bearing to protect early healing of labral refixation; (2) weight bearing as tolerated with transition to light activity; and (3) lifted restrictions to restore full strength and range of motion.
- In general athletes should expect a return to sport in 4 to 6 months after hip preservation surgery.
- Athletes should expect a high rate of return to play (87%) and return to level of competition (82%).
- Athletes with discrete chondral lesions treated with microfracture surgery have comparable rates of return to play.

INTRODUCTION

Background

Femoroacetabular impingement (FAI) is a pathologic mechanical process of the hip joint by which morphologic abnormalities of the acetabulum and/or femur, combined with vigorous hip motion, leads to repetitive collisions that result in damage to local soft-tissue structures.[1,2] There are 2 types of lesions described: the pincer lesion, which is defined as a local or global acetabular over-coverage, and the cam lesion, which is defined as a loss of the normal femoral head sphericity at the head-neck junction. In reality, the most common scenario likely involves a combination of the 2.[3]

Damage to the hip labrum, a fibrocartilaginous structure that lines the acetabular rim to help deepen the socket and helps provide joint stability, is common and leads to pain and instability. The articular hyaline cartilage, which lines the surface of the acetabulum and femur also is commonly affected. Such damage, directly and indirectly due to the resulting local chronic inflammatory state, is now recognized as a primary cause of idiopathic hip osteoarthritis (OA), leading to eventual destruction of the joint and need for total hip arthroplasty.[4] FAI is now recognized as one of the most common causes of hip pain, particularly in young and active patients. This is problematic for the elite athlete, because the symptoms of FAI often are debilitating, leading to decreased quality of life, suboptimal athletic performance, and even the inability to continue participation.

Surgical intervention in the form of femoroacetabular osteoplasty, by which the bony abnormalities leading to FAI are addressed, is widely performed and is now a potential option for athletes with promising results. This article provides a brief overview of FAI, including diagnosis and treatment, with particular focus on the athlete and return to play after femoroacetabular osteoplasty.

The Rothman Institute, Thomas Jefferson University, 925 Chestnut Street, Philadelphia, PA 19107, USA
* Corresponding author.
E-mail address: javadparvizi@gmail.com

Epidemiology

The true prevalence of FAI is largely unknown due to underdiagnosis and lack of consistent diagnostic criteria and because radiographic evidence of FAI does not necessarily translate to being symptomatic.[3] Evidence of radiographic FAI is widely prevalent in the United States. A systematic review done by Frank and colleagues[5] of 2114 hips found a prevalence of cam lesions, pincer lesions in 23.1% and 67% in the general population, respectively. In the athlete-specific cohort, cam lesions, pincer lesions were found at prevalence rates of 54.8% and 49.5%, respectively.[5] Furthermore radiographic cam lesions impingement is present in approximately half (49%) of patients with symptomatic hip joints according to a systematic review done by Mascarenhas and colleagues[6] In general, symptomatic cam lesions are more common in young, active men, whereas symptomatic pincer-type lesions predominate in middle-age women.[7]

Etiology

The etiology of FAI remains controversial but likely is multifactorial in nature.[4] The role of genetics has long been hypothesized but only recently investigated. Perhaps the best evidence for this comes from a siblings study by Pollard and colleagues[8]; 64 patients with FAI were enrolled and their siblings were compared with a spouse control group. Siblings were found to have increased risks of 2.8 and 2.0 for having similar cam lesions and pincer lesions, respectively, on radiograph compared with the control group.[8] This study is limited by the fact that siblings, in particular those raised together, often are exposed to similar social/environmental factors.[3] To date, the evidence to support genetic transmission remains scarce, and further research is necessary to appropriately investigate its role.[3]

The leading etiologic theory on the development of cam lesions centers around the hypothesis that there is a period of critical development of the proximal femoral physis. During this time, around ages 10 to 14 in boys and 8 to 12 in girls, repetitive injury to the physis results in deformity.[9] This theory first was supported by Murray and Duncan,[10] who found a high prevalence of pistol grip deformities in athletes.[10] Multiple studies have provided further support, citing high prevalence of FAI in high-impact sports, such as ice hockey, football, basketball, and soccer, across all levels of competition.[11–20] Agricola and colleagues[14] prospectively followed 63 preprofessional soccer players (mean age,

14.43 years; range, 12–19 years) to investigate the presence of cam deformity over the period of physeal closure. In hips with an open physis, the prevalence of cam deformities increased from 2.1% to 17.7% at mean follow-up of 2.4 years; 84.1% were found to have a normal head-neck junction initially, deceasing to 43.3% over the same period of time. After physeal closure, there was no significant increase in prevalence or severity of cam deformities, supporting the critical time of development hypothesis and showing that new lesions are not formed after physeal closure.[14] Some radiographic studies have furthered this hypothesis by finding abnormal epiphyseal extension of the growth plate in patients with FAI as a potential pathophysiologic cause.[21,22] Beck and colleagues[23] previously had found that juxtaphyseal trauma leads to stimulation of endochondral ossification with thickening and extension of the epiphysis in an in vitro rabbit model, providing a biologic mechanism to support these claims.[23]

Much of the prior research on etiology has focused solely on the cam lesion. Unfortunately, there have been few studies investigating the cause of pincer lesions. This represents an area in need of future research.[2,3]

Pathophysiology

Cam lesions

In the cam lesion, there is a loss of sphericity at the head-neck junction (**Fig. 1**).[23] Lesions vary in terms of exact location and size, but typically the abnormal osseous prominence is most significant at the anterior and lateral aspects of the femoral neck. As the irregular femoral head rotates within the acetabulum through range of motion, particularly during hip flexion under significant axial loading forces, the cam lesion makes direct contact with the anterosuperior aspect of the acetabulum, causing progressive damage and delamination of the articular cartilage.[4] Similarly, the adjacent acetabular labrum is often impinged between the bony surfaces, resulting in degeneration and tears.[24]

Pincer-type lesions

In the pincer-type lesion, there is over-coverage of the femoral head by the anterior acetabular rim that is greater than normal (see **Fig. 1**). This can be localized, in cases of acetabular retroversion, or generalized, in cases of acetabular protrusio.[7] As a result, there is similar impingement of the acetabular labrum between the bony surfaces, causing tears and degeneration.[24] In cases of pincer-type lesions, the

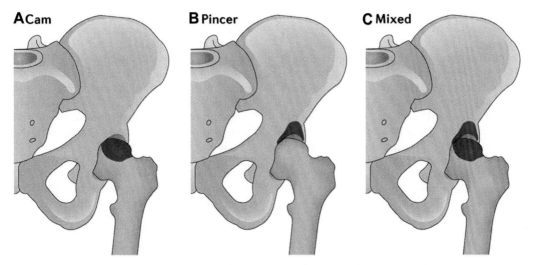

A Cam   **B** Pincer   **C** Mixed

Fig. 1. Illustration of cam-type and pincer-type lesions. (*From* Khan M, Bedi A, Fu F, et al. New perspectives on femoroacetabular impingement syndrome. Nat Rev Rheumatol 2016;12(5):303-10; with permission.)

pattern of articular cartilage damage can be in a coup-contrecoup fashion, with lesions present on the posteroinferior surface, due to migration of the femoral head within the acetabulum during flexion.[23]

As discussed previously, despite the different pathophysiology, the most frequent pathology is mixed cam lesions, pincer lesions deformity. Regardless of the mechanism, the chronic state of intra-articular damage leads to a localized inflammatory response, likely leading to further joint destruction.[24]

DISCUSSION
Diagnosis
Diagnosis of FAI can be quite challenging. A study done by Clohisy and colleagues[25] done in 2009 found that FAI patients were symptomatic for an average of 3.1 years before receiving a correct diagnosis. Patients in the study sought evaluation by an average of 4.2 health care providers prior to diagnosis, and inaccurate diagnoses were a common occurrence.[25] This is especially problematic given that multiple studies have reported longer length of preoperative symptomatic period to be a risk factor for worse outcomes after surgical intervention.[26] Increased awareness and appropriate clinical training likely would lead to improved outcomes and quality of life for patients suffering from FAI.

Unfortunately, diagnosis may be even more difficult in the athlete, due to higher likelihood of concurrent soft tissue injury related or unrelated to FAI at the time of symptom onset.[18] This is compounded by the fact that

radiographic evidence of FAI does not necessarily correlate with symptoms. Furthermore, hip pain often is poorly localized in nature, leading patients to have difficulty in accurately portraying their symptoms to clinicians.[2] For these reasons, diagnosis of FAI often is multifaceted and must be based on careful consideration of clinical presentation, physical examination, and diagnostic imaging.

Clinical Presentation
Patient history
Clinicians should inquire about any prior hip trauma or hip pathology. This includes developmental dysplasia of the hip, slipped capital femoral epiphysis, and Legg-Calvé-Perthes disease, because FAI can manifest as a late sequelae of all 3 even if surgically treated previously.[27]

In the athletic patient, specific consideration should be taken toward the type, intensity, and frequency of sport played. FAI is highly prevalent in athletes who participate in sports that require repetitive and excess joint loading during hip flexion, such as ice hockey, football, and basketball. Patients should be asked about specific exacerbating movements during sport.[28]

Symptomatology
Symptom onset often is insidious in nature. At first patients tend to experience pain only with exacerbating activity, often during heavy joint loading or quick rotation. Symptom severity typically then escalates and patients often begin to complain of pain throughout the day, exacerbated by even light activity, such as cleaning, walking up and down stairs, buying groceries,

and standing. Pain at nighttime with difficulty sleeping also is common as symptoms progress.[29]

Pain is located most frequently in the groin (88%) and lateral aspect of the hip over the greater trochanter (67%) (Fig. 2). Groin pain is typically deep and dull, with a C sign, in which the patient cups a hand over the groin and above the greater trochanter, classically described (Fig. 3).[25] Pain intensity can vary from mild to severe.[30] Patients also may experience pain in a variety of locations, including the buttock, lumbar spine, thigh, and knee. Other symptoms include stiffness, instability, hip clicking, popping, and catching.[24,27,31]

Physical Examination
Range of motion
Range of motion should be evaluated, in particular passive hip flexion and internal rotation. Wyss and colleagues[32] showed a strong association between the amount of internal rotation during 90° of flexion with the presence and extent of cam deformity in symptomatic and asymptomatic patients. Symptomatic patients tended to have more severe limitations, averaging only 4° of internal rotation, compared with 28° in the control group.[32] Hack and colleagues,[33] however, found that only 25% of patients with internal rotation of less than 20° actually had a cam lesions deformity on magnetic resonance imaging (MRI).[33] Thus, limited range of motion, like most physical examination findings for FAI, is considered a sensitive but not specific finding.

Provocative maneuvers
Provocative maneuvers serve 2 main goals: (1) to reproduce impingement by abutting the femur against the acetabulum during range of motion, in cases of the FADDIR, FABER, and posterior impingement tests; and (2) to localize whether or not pain is resulting from an intra-articular source, in cases of the Stinchfield and log roll tests.[27] Pain elicited by each of the following provocative maneuvers is considered a positive finding:

- FADDIR (flexion, adduction, internal rotation)—the hip is placed in passive flexion at 90°. The hip then is adducted and internally rotated (Fig. 4).

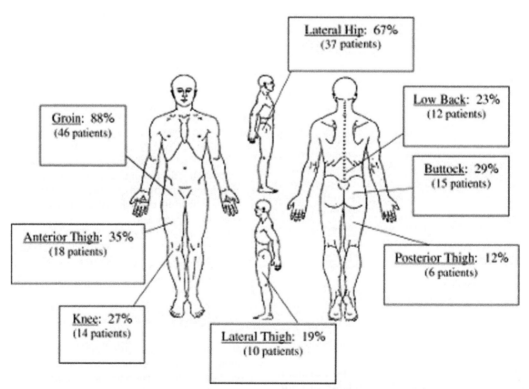

Fig. 2. Distribution of pain in symptomatic FAI patients reported in a study. (*From* "Clohisy JC, Knaus ER, Hunt DM, et al. Clinical presentation of patients with symptomatic anterior hip impingement. Clin Orthop. 2009;467:638-644.")

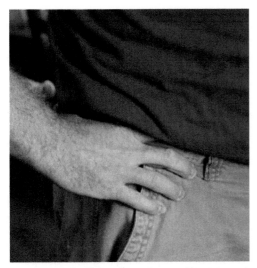

Fig. 3. Example of the classic C sign of hip joint pain. (*From* "Rimmasch A, Ravert P. Femoroacetabular Impingement: A Guide to Diagnosis in Primary Care. The Journal for Nurse Practitioners. 2013;9(9):606-611.")

- FABER (flexion, abduction, external rotation)—the hip is placed in passive flexion at 90°. The hip then is abducted and externally rotated (**Fig. 5**).
- Posterior impingement test—the hip is placed in extension and external rotation.
- Stinchfield—while supine, the hip is flexed against resistance
- Log roll—while supine, the thigh is gently rotated internally and externally.

Unfortunately, provocative maneuvers are limited in their diagnostic utility for FAI. Martin and colleagues[31] found FADDIR and FABER tests to have sensitivities of 78% and 60%, respectively, and specificities of only 10% and 18%, respectively.[31] A meta-analysis by Reiman and colleagues[34] found only the FADDIR examination to be supported by enough evidence for screening purposes. All other physical examination maneuvers lack high-quality evidence to be relied on for FAI.[34]

Gait and posture

Careful consideration of patient gait should be taken. Compensatory extra-articular disorders are a common finding in FAI, often leading to weakened abductor muscle strength and a Trendelenburg gait or lateral lurch. Attention should be made to patient posture during the examination. Impingement often is exacerbated by flexion of the hip. As a result, many patients classically adjust their seated posture to a slouch in an attempt to alleviate pain.[27]

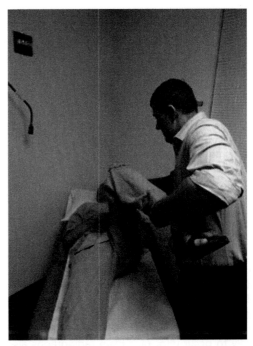

Fig. 4. FADDIR physical examination maneuver. (*From* "Rimmasch A, Ravert P. Femoroacetabular Impingement: A Guide to Diagnosis in Primary Care. The Journal for Nurse Practitioners. 2013;9(9):606-611.")

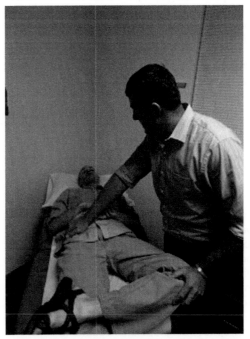

Fig. 5. FABER physical examination maneuver. (*From* "Rimmasch A, Ravert P. Femoroacetabular Impingement: A Guide to Diagnosis in Primary Care. The Journal for Nurse Practitioners. 2013;9(9):606-611.")

Imaging

Imaging modalities often used in the work-up of FAI include radiography, MRI, and magnetic resonance (MR) arthrogram, ultrasound, and computed tomography (CT).

Radiography

Imaging assessment typically begins with radiography. An anteroposterior view allowing visualization of both hips is important. This allows for assessment of hip symmetry, evidence of acetabular retroversion, and developmental dysplasia of the hip. Anteroposterior images should be supplemented by at least 1 additional view, often the frog-leg lateral, cross-table lateral, Dunn lateral, or false-profile. The most common location of cam lesions is anterolateral. Frog-leg lateral, cross-table latearal, Dunn lateral, or false-profile allow for the assessment of femoral head-neck offset and measurement of the alpha angle, classically used to grade the presence and severity of cam-lesions deformity, in each plane that impingement is most likely to occur (Fig. 6).[35] Plain radiographs also help rule out other osseous pathology, such as stress fractures, and help quantify the presence and severity of preexisting OA of the hip.

Magnetic resonance imaging and magnetic resonance arthrogram

After plain radiographs, MRI often is the next imaging step in the diagnostic work-up of FAI. This is because MRI possesses a superior to ability to identify and assess the extent of damage to soft tissue structures around and within the hip. An accuracy of as high as 90% can be attained in diagnosis of a labral tear (Fig. 7).[36] Tears of the articular cartilage and evidence of OA often can be identified on MRI.

MR arthrograms allow for the addition of localized gadolinium contrast via intra-articular injection, frequently done under fluoroscopic guidance. The contrast fluid also serves to distend the joint space itself and help better visualize labral and cartilage tears.[27,36]

Identification of a labral tear on MRI, however, does not guarantee it to be the source of a patients' symptoms. Martin and colleagues[31] found that in 47 patients with definite or possible labral tears on MRI arthrogram, 45% did not achieve a greater than 50% reduction in pain after intra-articular anesthetic injection.[31] For this reason it is important to correlate imaging findings with the clinical picture to reach the appropriate diagnosis and treatment.[35]

Ultrasound

Ultrasound can play an important role in the diagnosis of hip pain, particularly in athletes. It is possible to identify labral and chondral injury via ultrasound, albeit with lower accuracy (44%) compared with MR arthrography due to incomplete visualization and its user-dependent nature (Fig. 8).[37] Instead the strength of ultrasound lies in its ability to dynamically assess the hip. Specifically, patients can be brought through painful range of motion to identify impingement and other common causes of sport-related hip pain, such as iliopsoas bursitis and iliopsoas tendinitis.[35]

Computed topography

CT provides 3-dimensional modeling and optimal characterization of the osseous structures of the hip. CT imaging allows for detailed topography of both cam and pincer deformities, which may aid in preoperative planning (Fig. 9).[24] Compared with plain radiographs, however, the greater cost, time, and radiation exposure outweigh the minimal added information it provides.[35] Although newer, low-contrast techniques are being pioneered, CT currently is not a recommended routine imaging modality.

Image-guided injections

Fluoroscopic or ultrasound image-guided injections can help provide valuable information in the work-up of sport-related hip pain and FAI. Intra-articular injections of local anesthetic can help localize pain to an intra-articular source.[38] A positive response to intra-articular injection also is a prognostic indicator for successful outcome after surgical intervention for the treatment of FAI.[39] If there are signs of an extraarticular pain source on examination or imaging, anesthetic and corticosteroid injection of local structures can be done.

Treatment
Nonsurgical

The most effective nonoperative treatment of FAI is activity modification. For an athlete, this includes avoidance of any specific sports demands that exacerbate symptoms. Emara and colleagues[40] prospectively studied 37 patients who were instructed to modify activities of daily living to limit range of motion and joint loading and found significant improvement in function and symptom scores.[40] Understandably, for young, active patients wishing to return to normal activity or high-level athletics, doing so may not be desirable or even feasible. The benefits of activity modification also are short-lived, and symptom exacerbation likely occur once an athlete returns to the high physical demand of their sport.

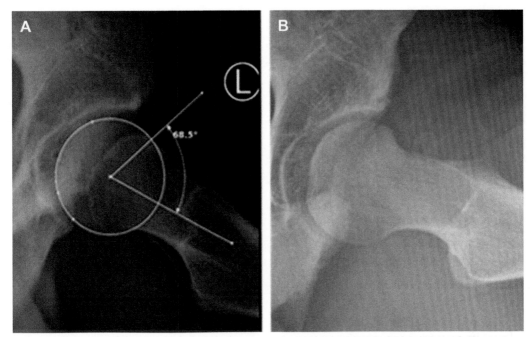

Fig. 6. Modified Dunn lateral view of left hip in 16-year-old male patient with cam deformity. (A) Alpha angle. (B) Modified Dunn lateral after cam resection. (From "Griffin JW, Weber AE, Kuhns B, Lewis P, Nho SJ. Imaging in Hip Arthroscopy for Femoroacetabular Impingement. Clinics in Sports Medicine. 2016;35(3):331-344.")

Other nonoperative treatment modalities include physiotherapy, nonsteroidal anti-inflammatory drugs, and intra-articular joint injections. Physical therapy typically involves exercise focused on hip and core strength and mobility.[2] Anesthetic, hyaluronic acid, and corticosteroid intra-articular hip injections also have been used in certain circumstances. Khan and colleagues[39] noted that injections, particularly with hyaluronic acid, showed therapeutic benefit at 12 months.[39] Caution should be taken when using corticosteroid injections, however, due to their cytotoxic effect on chondrocytes and association with accelerating joint deterioration.[41,42]

There is a paucity of data comparing outcomes of nonsurgical and surgical treatment of symptomatic FAI. A systematic review by Wall and colleagues[43] in 2013 on the nonoperative

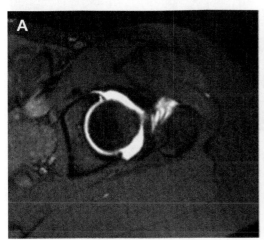
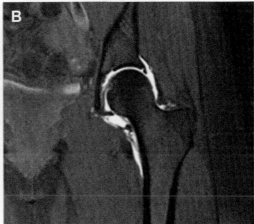

Fig. 7. (A) Axial and (B) coronal MR arthrograms demonstrating an anterolateral labral tear of the left hip. (From "Griffin JW, Weber AE, Kuhns B, Lewis P, Nho SJ. Imaging in Hip Arthroscopy for Femoroacetabular Impingement. Clinics in Sports Medicine. 2016;35(3):331-344.")

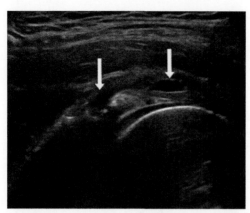

Fig. 8. Right acetabular labral tear with irregular anechoic acetabular paralabral cysts (arrows). (*From* "Gao G, Fu Q, Cui L, Xu Y. The Diagnostic Value of Ultrasound in Anterosuperior Acetabular Labral Tear. Arthroscopy: The Journal of Arthroscopic & Related Surgery. 2019;35(9):2591-2597.")

treatment of FAI reported that the majority of the literature promoting nonoperative treatment and physical therapy is based mostly on opinion, and clinical evidence to support nonoperative treatment was weak and should be viewed with caution.[43] More recently in 2019, Ayeni[44] reported on a randomized controlled trial on 348 patients who were randomized to hip arthroscopy or standard outpatient physiotherapy. At 12 months, hip arthroscopy improved hip-related quality of life compared with personalized hip therapy.[44] As stated previously, several studies have reported that patients with longer preoperative symptom periods have worse outcomes after surgery.[45] In addition, delayed correction of FAI may lead to greater chondral damage and disease progression. For this reason, in young, athletic surgical candidates with little evidence of preexisting arthritis, surgical correction should be considered the definitive treatment of choice at this moment.

Surgical

First described by Ganz and colleagues,[46] the surgical treatment of FAI serves 2 main purposes: (1) to improve pain and function of the joint and (2) possibly delay or prevent the progression of joint arthrosis.[4,46]

Approach

Surgical treatment of FAI can be performed via 3 main approaches: open surgical dislocation, anterior miniopen, and arthroscopic. It is recommended that the choice of surgical approach is dictated primarily by the specific bony deformity and intra-articular pathology.[47] For example, open hip surgery generally is reserved for correction of more complex bony abnormalities.[48] Positive short-term and midterm outcomes have been reported on all 3 techniques, with improvement in pain and function, low failure rates, and minimal complications.[49–55] Open

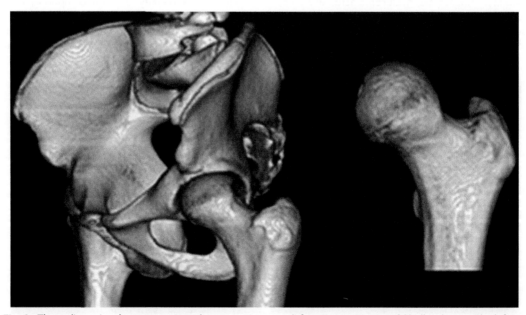

Fig. 9. Three-dimensional reconstructions demonstrating cam deformity in a 16-year-old ballet dancer. The left image is the reconstruction of the entire pelvis and the right image is the reconstruction of the femur bone alone. (*From* "Griffin JW, Weber AE, Kuhns B, Lewis P, Nho SJ. Imaging in Hip Arthroscopy for Femoroacetabular Impingement. Clinics in Sports Medicine. 2016;35(3):331-344.")

surgical dislocation allows for optimal visualization of the joint but requires major soft tissue intervention and has been noted to have a comparatively higher major complication rate. The miniopen method is less invasive, does not require traction, and allows for dynamic testing of range of motion intraoperatively but has a significant incidence of iatrogenic injury to the lateral femoral cutaneous nerve.[56] The arthroscopic method provides complete visualization of the joint, but requires traction and is technically demanding, with high rates of initial complications and revision rates for incomplete correction of bony deformities, causing impingement for inexperienced surgeons.[47] Given the widespread popularity of the arthroscopic technique and its minimally invasive nature that portends quicker return to play, however, it tends to be the approach of choice for most athletes.[57]

Postoperative rehabilitation

There is no universal postoperative protocol after surgical treatment of FAI in the athlete. Instead, recovery varies based on several factors, including extent of pathology, specific surgical intervention performed, type of sport, and level of competition.[58] For simple labral débridement and recontouring of the acetabular rim, athletes can resume weight-bearing status as tolerated immediately postoperatively. If the labrum is refixed, the repair site should be protected during the early healing phase with toe-touch weight bearing and limited range of motion. Flexion should be limited to 90° flexion with only minimal internal/external rotation. Protected weightbearing should be maintained for 3 weeks to 6 weeks.[58] In cases of femoral head-neck osteoplasty for osseous cam lesions, the most common bony pathology in the young athlete, patients should avoid any twisting movements for 4 weeks. This is because of the unlikely but potentially devastating complication of femoral neck fracture.[51] In the second phase of rehabilitation, after initial restrictions are lifted and patients have regained adequate motor control, light activities are permitted. These include activities of daily living and low-impact exercise. This second phase still requires restriction of high-impact/twisting activities and typically last 3 months, during which full bony remodeling takes place. One caveat is that, in cases of microfracture performed for full-thickness chondral tears, athletes typically are restricted to partial weight bearing for 2 months to optimize healing of the fibrocartilage response. At 3 months, restrictions are lifted and athletes are able to progress as tolerated.

At this point, rehabilitation progression is variable but typically requires an additional 1 months to 3 months.[24,58] This depends on multiple patient factors, including type of sport and level of competition. In total, athletes should expect a return to sport after hip preservation surgery in 4 months to 6 months.[59]

Outcomes

Several studies have reported on rates of return to play after hip preservation surgery in the athlete. Philippon and colleagues[60] reported on a total of 45 professional athletes who underwent arthroscopic treatment of FAI and found 93% resumed play at some point. This number, however, did decline to 78% over a follow-up period of 1.6 years.[60] Philippon and colleagues[61] then later examined 28 elite hockey players who underwent arthroscopic treatment of FAI and found a high level of patient satisfaction and return to skating and hockey drills at an average of 3.4 months.[61] Byrd[58] studied a cohort of 172 athletes across all levels of competition treated for FAI arthroscopically; 89% of professional athletes and 90% of intercollegiate athletes were able to return to their previous level of competition at 1-year follow-up.[58] Nho and colleagues[62] studied outcomes in 47 elite-level athletes among varsity high school, college, and professional levels. Similarly, 92.3% of athletes reported return to play at the same level of competition, with 78% of athletes continuing play at 1-year follow-up and 73% at 2-year follow-up. Significant improvement in functional outcome scores were noted in their study.[62] This level of consistency and high rate of return to sport also was confirmed by a systematic review by Casartelli and colleagues[47] that found that among 977 athletes across all levels of competition, 87% returned to sport, with 82% returning to the same level of sport as before the onset of FAI symptoms.[47]

Additional Factors
Microfracture surgery

There is some preliminary evidence to show that athletes who require microfracture surgery for discrete full-thickness articular cartilage tears have favorable outcomes. McDonald and colleagues[63] studied 39 athletes with microfracture and compared them to 94 without microfracture and found comparable rates of return to play and continued play at 3-year follow-up.[63]

Level of competition

Many studies have previously reported rates of return to play to be higher in professionals compared with amateur and collegiate athletes.[38,64] These findings likely are biased by multiple confounding factors, however, including socioeconomic pressure and greater access to medical care for professional athletes. More recently, several studies have shown comparably high rates of return to play (84%–93%), and return to same level of competition (74%–89%).[65–67]

In general, there is a large body of evidence to suggest that athletes who are candidates for hip preservation surgery should expect to return to sport at a high rate across all levels of competition.[68]

Words of Caution

Not all patients experience positive outcomes after several risk factors for less optimal outcomes have been cited, including older age, longer preoperative symptomatic period, higher body mass index, prior hip surgery, presence of hip dysplasia or acetabular retroversion, and, most importantly, level of preoperative joint arthritis.[26,69] Athletes with diffuse hip OA at the time of surgery may never be able to return to play. Even under ideal circumstances, some athletes may never return to play or regain the sporting abilities they once had. Return to sport does not necessarily equate to high satisfaction or full recovery of sporting ability either. Additional studies are needed to determine the effect of symptomatic FAI and hip preservation surgery on sport-specific skills.

Return to sport after hip preservation surgery may not always be in the best interest of the athlete either. High-impact sport activities potentially may accelerate the degenerative process.[47] Patients with significant chondral lesions and evidence of joint arthrosis should proceed with caution and highly consider lifetime activity modification to preserve the joint. For these reasons, it is vital that clinicians set realistic expectations with patients and thoroughly explain the nature of FAI and hip OA.

SUMMARY

FAI is a condition that results from a mismatch of congruency between the femoral head and the acetabulum. This condition is most common among young, active patients and may lead to pain, decreased quality of life, and an inability to participate in athletics. Hip preservation surgery is widely performed now and is a definite treatment option for athletes at all levels of competition. In general, athletes have reported high rates of return to play and satisfaction and

should expect rehabilitation to require approximately 4 months to 6 months.

CLINIC CARE POINTS

- Diagnosis of FAI is multifaceted. Careful consideration of clinical presentation, physical examination, and diagnostic imaging is necessary to reach the correct diagnosis.
- Rehabilitation protocol for the athlete consists of 3 main phases: (1) partial weight bearing to protect early healing of labral refixation with a focus on recovery of passive hip range of motion; (2) weight bearing as tolerated with transition to light activity for improvement of neuromuscular function; and (3) lifted restrictions to restore full strength, range of motion, and motor control for sport-specific tasks.[24,58]
- In general, athletes should expect a return to sport after hip preservation surgery in 4 months to 6 months.[59]
- Athletes should expect a high rate of return to play (87%) and return to level of competition (82%).[47]
- Athletes with discrete chondral lesions treated with microfracture surgery have comparable rates of return to play.[63]
- The level of sport-specific skills that are recovered after hip preservation surgery is unknown and further studies are necessary.
- Patients with significant preoperative arthritis tend to have worse outcomes, and return to high-impact sporting activities may accelerate the degenerative process in such cases.[47]

DISCLOSURE

This research was funded by The Rothman Institute and Thomas Jefferson University.

REFERENCES

1. Sankar WN, Nevitt M, Parvizi J, et al. Femoroacetabular impingement: defining the condition and its role in the pathophysiology of osteoarthritis. J Am Acad Orthop Surg 2013;21:S7–15.
2. Egger AC, Frangiamore S, Rosneck J. Femoroacetabular Impingement. Sports Med Arthrosc Rev 2016;24(4):e53–8.
3. Packer JD, Safran MR. The etiology of primary femoroacetabular impingement: genetics or acquired deformity? J Hip Preserv Surg 2015;2:249–57.

4. Ganz R, Parvizi J, Beck M, et al. Femoroacetabular impingement: a cause for osteoarthritis of the hip. Clin Orthop 2003;417:112–20.

5. Frank JM, Harris JD, Erickson BJ, et al. Prevalence of femoroacetabular impingement imaging findings in asymptomatic volunteers: a systematic review. Arthroscopy 2015;31(6):1199–204.

6. Mascarenhas VV, Rego P, Dantas P, et al. Imaging prevalence of femoroacetabular impingement in symptomatic patients, athletes, and asymptomatic individuals: A systematic review. Eur J Radiol 2016;85(1):73–95.

7. Ganz R, Leunig M, Leunig-Ganz K, et al. The etiology of osteoarthritis of the hip. Clin Orthop 2008;466:264–72.

8. Pollard TC, Villar RN, Norton MR, et al. Genetic influences in the aetiology of femoroacetabular impingement: a sibling study. J Bone Joint Surg Br 2010;92:209–16.

9. Johnson AC, Shaman MA, Ryan TG. Femoroacetabular impingement in former high-level youth soccer players. Am J Sports Med 2012;40(6):1342–6.

10. Murray RO, Duncan C. Athletic activity in adolescence as an etiological factor in degenerative hip disease. J Bone Joint Surg Br 1971;53:406–19.

11. Siebenrock K, Ferner F, Noble P, et al. The cam-type deformity of the proximal femur arises in childhood in response to vigorous sporting activity. Clin Orthop Relat Res 2011;469:3229–40.

12. Siebenrock KA, Kaschka I, Frauchiger L, et al. Prevalence of cam-type deformity and hip pain in elite ice hockey players before and after the end of growth. Am J Sports Med 2013;41:2308–13.

13. Philippon MJ, Ho CP, Briggs KK, et al. Prevalence of increased alpha angles as a measure of cam-type femoroacetabular impingement in youth ice hockey players. Am J Sports Med 2013;41:1357–62.

14. Agricola R, Heijboer MP, Ginai AZ, et al. A cam deformity is gradually acquired during skeletal maturation in adolescent and young male soccer players: A prospective study with minimum 2-year follow-up. Am J Sports Med 2014;42:798–806.

15. Nepple JJ, Vigdorchik JM, Clohisy JC. What is the association between sports participation and the development of proximal femoral cam deformity? A systematic review and meta-analysis. Am J Sports Med 2015;43:2833–40.

16. Gerhardt MB, Romero AA, Silvers HJ, et al. The prevalence of radiographic hip abnormalities in elite soccer players. Am J Sports Med 2012;40:584–8.

17. Silvis ML, Mosher TJ, Smetana BS, et al. High prevalence of pelvic and hip magnetic resonance imaging findings in asymptomatic collegiate and professional hockey players. Am J Sports Med 2011;39:715–21.

18. Jackson TJ, Starkey C, McElhiney D, et al. Epidemiology of hip injuries in the national basketball association: a 24-year overview. Orthop J Sports Med 2013;1. 2325967113499130.

19. Nepple JJ, Brophy RH, Matava MJ, et al. Radiographic findings of femoroacetabular impingement in national football league combine athletes undergoing radiographs for previous hip or groin pain. Arthroscopy 2012;28:1396–403.

20. Larson CM, Sikka RS, Sardelli MC, et al. Increasing alpha angle is predictive of athletic-related "hip" and "groin" pain in collegiate national football league prospects. Arthroscopy 2013;29:405–10.

21. Siebenrock K, Wahab KA, Werlen S, et al. Abnormal extension of the femoral head epiphysis as a cause of cam impingement. Clin Orthop 2004;418:54–60.

22. Siebenrock KA, Behning A, Mamisch TC, et al. Growth plate alteration precedes cam-type deformity in elite basketball players. Clin Orthop Relat Res 2013;471:1084–91.

23. Beck M, Kalhor M, Leunig M, et al. Hip morphology influences the pattern of damage to the acetabular cartilage: femoroacetabular impingement as a cause of early osteoarthritis of the hip. J Bone Joint Surg Br 2005;87:1012–8.

24. Macfarlane RJ, Haddad FS. The diagnosis and management of femoro-acetabular impingement. Ann R Coll Surg Engl 2010;92:363–7.

25. Clohisy JC, Knaus ER, Hunt DM, et al. Clinical presentation of patients with symptomatic anterior hip impingement. Clin Orthop 2009;467:638–44.

26. Saadat E, Martin SD, Thornhill TS, et al. Factors associated with the failure of surgical treatment for femoroacetabular impingement: review of the literature. Am J Sports Med 2014;42:1487–95.

27. Nepple JJ, Prather H, Trousdale RT, et al. Clinical diagnosis of femoroacetabular impingement. J Am Acad Orthop Surg 2013;21:S16–9.

28. Parvaresh KC, Wichman D, Rasio J, et al. Return to sport after femoroacetabular impingement surgery and sport-specific considerations: a comprehensive review. Curr Rev Musculoskelet Med 2020;13(3):213–9.

29. Burnett RS, Della Rocca GJ, Prather H, et al. Clinical presentation of patients with tears of the acetabular labrum. J Bone Joint Surg Am 2006;88:1448–57.

30. Byrd JWT. Physical examination. In: Byrd JWT, editor. Operative hip arthroscopy. 2nd edition. New York: Springer; 2005. p. 36–50.

31. Martin RL, Irrgang JJ, Sekiya JK. The diagnostic accuracy of a clinical examination in determining intra-articular hip pain for potential hip arthroscopy candidates. Arthroscopy 2008;24:1013–8.

32. Wyss TF, Clark JM, Weishaupt D, et al. Correlation between internal rotation and bony anatomy in the hip. Clin Orthop Relat Res 2007;460:152–8.

33. Hack K, Di Primio GD, Rakhra K, et al. Prevalence of cam-type   femoroacetabular   impingement

morphology in asymptomatic volunteers. J Bone Joint Surg Am 2010;92(14):2436–44.

34. Reiman MP, Goode AP, Cook CE, et al. Diagnostic accuracy of clinical tests for the diagnosis of hip femoroacetabular impingement/labral tear: a systematic review with meta-analysis. Br J Sports Med 2015;49:811–23.

35. Jacobson JA, Bedi A, Sekiya JK, et al. Evaluation of the painful athletic hip: Imaging options and imaging-guided injections. Am J Roentgenol 2012;199:516–24.

36. Perdikakis E, Karachalios T, Katonis P, et al. Comparison of MR-arthrography and MDCT-arthrography for detection of labral and articular cartilage hip pathology. Skeletal Radiol 2011; 40(11):1441–7.

37. Troelsen A, Jacobsen S, Bolvig L, et al. Ultrasound versus magnetic resonance arthrography in acetabular labral tear diagnostics: a prospective comparison in 20 dysplastic hips. Acta Radiol 2007;48(9): 1004–10.

38. Byrd JW, Jones KS. Arthroscopic management of femoroacetabular impingement in athletes. Am J Sports Med 2011;39(Suppl 1):7S–13S.

39. Khan W, Khan M, Alradwan H, et al. Utility of intra-articular hip injections for femoroacetabular impingement: a systematic review. Orthop J Sports Med 2015;3. 2325967115601030.

40. Emara K, Samir W, Motasem EH, et al. Conservative treatment for mild femoroacetabular impingement. J Orthop Surg 2011;19:41–5.

41. Fubini SL, Todhunter RJ, Burton-Wurster N, et al. Corticosteroids alter the differentiated phenotype of articular chondrocytes. J Orthop Res 2001; 19(4):688–95.

42. Dragoo JL, Braun HJ, Kim HJ, et al. The in vitro chondrotoxicity of single-dose local anesthetics. Am J Sports Med 2012;40(4):794–9.

43. Wall PD, Fernandez M, Griffin DR, et al. Nonoperative treatment for femoroacetabular impingement: a systematic review of the literature. PM R 2013;5:418–26.

44. Ayeni OR. In femoroacetabular impingement syndrome, hip arthroscopy improved hip-related quality of life at 12 months compared with conservative care. J Bone Joint Surg 2019;101(4):371.

45. Kunze KN, Beck EC, Nwachukwu BU, et al. Early hip arthroscopy for femoroacetabular impingement syndrome provides superior outcomes when compared with delaying surgical treatment beyond 6 months. Am J Sports Med 2019;47(9):2038–44.

46. Ganz R, Gill TJ, Gautier E, et al. Surgical dislocation of the adult hip. J Bone Joint Surg Br 2001;83-B(8): 1119–24.

47. Casartelli NC, Leunig M, Maffiuletti NA, et al. Return to sport after hip surgery for femoroacetabular impingement: a systematic review. Br J Sports Med 2015;49:819–24.

48. Zaltz I, Kelly BT, Larson CM, et al. Surgical treatment of femoroacetabular impingement: what are the limits of hip arthroscopy? Arthroscopy 2014; 30(1):99–110.

49. Parvizi J, Huang R, Diaz-Ledezma C, et al. Mini-open femoroacetabular osteoplasty: how do these patients do? J Arthroplasty 2012;27(8 suppl):122–5.

50. Peters CL, Erickson JA. Treatment of femoroacetabular impingement with surgical dislocation and debridement in young adults. J Bone Joint Surg Am 2006;88:1735–41.

51. Sampson TG. Complications of hip arthroscopy. Clin Sports Med 2001;20:831–5.

52. Scher DL, Belmont PJ Jr, Owens BD. Osteonecrosis of the femoral head after hip arthroscopy. Clin Orthop Relat Res 2010;468:3121–5.

53. Lee J-W, Hwang D-S, Kang C, et al. Arthroscopic repair of acetabular labral tears associated with femoroacetabular impingement: 7–10 years of long-term follow-up results. Clin Orthop Surg 2019;11(1):28.

54. Beck M, Leunig M, Parvizi J, et al. Anterior femoroacetabular impingement: part II. Midterm results of surgical treatment. Clin Orthop 2004;418:67–73.

55. Cohen SB, Huang R, Ciccotti MG, et al. Treatment of femoroacetabular impingement in athletes using a mini-direct anterior approach. Am J Sports Med 2012;40:1620–7.

56. Botser I, Jackson T, Smith T, et al. Open surgical dislocation versus arthroscopic treatment of femoroacetabular impingement. Am J Orthop 2014;43: 209–14.

57. Nwachukwu BU, Rebolledo BJ, McCormick F, et al. Arthroscopic versus open treatment of femoroacetabular impingement: a systematic review of medium- to long-term outcomes. Am J Sports Med 2016;44:1062–8.

58. Byrd JW. Femoroacetabular impingement in athletes, part II: treatment and outcomes. Sports Health 2010;2:403–9.

59. Voight ML, Robinson K, Gill L, et al. Postoperative rehabilitation guidelines for hip arthroscopy in an active population. Sports Health 2010;2:222–30.

60. Philippon M, Schenker M, Briggs K, et al. Femoroacetabular impingement in 45 professional athletes: associated pathologies and return to sport following arthroscopic decompression. Knee Surg Sports Traumatol Arthrosc 2007;15:908–14.

61. Philippon MJ, Weiss DR, Kuppersmith DA, et al. Arthroscopic labral repair and treatment of femoroacetabular impingement in professional hockey players. Am J Sports Med 2010;38:99–104.

62. Nho SJ, Magennis EM, Singh CK, et al. Outcomes after the arthroscopic treatment of femoroacetabular impingement in a mixed group of high-level athletes. Am J Sports Med 2011;39(suppl):14S–19SS.

63. McDonald JE, Herzog MM, Philippon MJ. Return to play after hip arthroscopy with microfracture in elite athletes. Arthroscopy 2013;29:330–5.

64. Malviya A, Paliobeis CP, Villar RN. Do professional athletes perform better than recreational athletes after arthroscopy for femoroacetabular impingement? Clin Orthop Relat Res 2013;471: 2477–83.

65. Litrenta J, Mu BH, Ortiz-Declet V, et al. Hip arthroscopy successfully treats femoroacetabular impingement in adolescent athletes. J Pediatr Orthop 2020; 40(3):e156–60. https://doi.org/10.1097/BPO. 0000000000001411.

66. Weber AE, Kuhns BD, Cvetanovich GL, et al. Amateur and recreational athletes return to sport at a high rate following hip arthroscopy for femoroacetabular impingement. Arthroscopy 2017; 33(4):748–55.

67. Mohan R, Johnson NR, Hevesi M, et al. Return to sport and clinical outcomes after hip arthroscopic labral repair in young amateur athletes: minimum 2-year follow-up. Arthroscopy 2017; 33(9):1679–84.

68. Alradwan H, Philippon MJ, Farrokhyar F, et al. Return to preinjury activity levels after surgical management of femoroacetabular impingement in athletes. Arthroscopy 2012;28:1567–76.

69. Ceylan HH, Vahedi H, Azboy I, et al. Mini-open femoroacetabular osteoplasty. J Bone Joint Surg 2020;102(12):e59.

Allowed Activities After Primary Total Knee Arthroplasty and Total Hip Arthroplasty

Wissam S. Fawaz, MD, Bassam A. Masri, MD, FRCSC*

KEYWORDS

- Total hip arthroplasty • Total knee arthroplasty • Activities • Joint loading • Return to sport
- Return to work

KEY POINTS

- Patients' expectations from total joint replacement (TJR) surpass pain control and quality of life to include sports and athletic activities.
- Wear rate is a function of activity level and joint loading.
- Patient preoperative counseling is essential to keep realistic expectations and to prevent disappointment.
- Physician recommendations are becoming more lenient toward low and moderate impact activities with remaining controversy toward most high impact sports.
- Most TJR patients are able to return to work, fewer are able to return to sports (RTS), especially those with several confounding variables including gender, age, body mass index, comorbidities, and preoperative activity level.

INTRODUCTION

Lack of physical activity is one of the most important modifiable risk factors leading to major chronic noncommunicable diseases including obesity, cardiovascular disease, type 2 diabetes mellitus, hypertension, osteoporosis, and depression.[1,2] The relationship between regular exercise and cardiovascular health has been substantially proven over the years and its effect on the reduction of overall mortality and morbidity.[3] With the increasing life expectancy in North America, there is a parallel increase in the number of individuals suffering from painful osteoarthritis that limits their physical activity and active lifestyle.

In Canada, by 2031, it is estimated that the number of 45 to 64 year olds diagnosed with osteoarthritis will double to reach almost 2.1 million (compared with 1991).[4] Total joint replacement (TJR) remains, the best therapeutic option for symptomatic and debilitating end-stage osteoarthritis. According to the American Joint Registry, the number of primary total hip arthroplasty (THA) is projected to grow by 71%, reaching 635,000 procedures by 2030 in the United States. Similarly, the number of primary total knee arthroplasty (TKA) is projected to grow by 85%, reaching 1.26 million procedures by 2030.[5]

Historically, pain relief and gain of function have been the main expected outcomes of TJR. However, patients are increasingly seeking a more active lifestyle, trying to return to their previous levels of activity, even trying to reach a certain level of athletic abilities that they used to possess before the onset of osteoarthritis symptoms.[6]

Department of Orthopaedic Surgery, University of British Columbia, Complex Joint Clinic, Third Floor, 2775 Laurel Street, Vancouver, British Columbia V5Z 1M9, Canada
* Corresponding author.
E-mail address: bas.masri@ubc.ca

Orthop Clin N Am 51 (2020) 441–452
https://doi.org/10.1016/j.ocl.2020.06.002
0030-5898/20/© 2020 Elsevier Inc. All rights reserved.

Despite the overwhelming evidence regarding the benefits of regular exercise on reduction of mortality/morbidity and incidence of chronic diseases, it comes with the price of increasing the risk of implant wear and loosening potential with possibly higher revision rates. In the literature, little evidence describes the direct effect of recreational and athletic activity on TJR outcomes.

This article reviews the evidence in the literature that best describes the allowed general and sports activities after primary THA and TKA. Although it is difficult, the goal is to find the balance between reaching the necessary level of physical activity for a healthy lifestyle, meeting the expectations of a more demanding population, and preserving at the same time the survival of the implanted prosthetic joints, which is important for the continued success of total joint arthroplasty.

CURRENT EVIDENCE
Wear and Level of Activity After Total Joint Replacement
Following TJR, each step releases up to 500,000 submicron-sized polyethylene particles.[7] These particles activate macrophages that release cytokines, such as tumor necrosis factor-α, interleukin-1, prostaglandin E_2, and others, which are responsible for osteolysis and aseptic loosening of prosthetic implants.[8] Factors that contribute to polyethylene wear are divided into surgical technique-related, material properties-related, and patients-related. Our focus in this article is mainly on patient-related factors.

According to Kuster and Stachowiak[9] the volume of wear particles is linearly proportional to the number of steps and exponentially proportional to the applied force (joint loading) and surface roughness.

There is no doubt that the activity level (thus wear) varies to a certain extent with age. However, several studies have shown that the walking distance/number of steps correlates weakly with chronologic age. Two studies showed similar levels of activity between a young and an old population following primary TKA,[10,11] whereby patients undergoing TKA (641,305 steps/year) were significantly less active than patients undergoing THA (947,905 steps/year) with minimal correlation with age.[12] In the year 2000, a John Charnley Award–winning study proved that wear is a function of use. Walking was the most common activity of the studied population. The study showed that for a 70-kg patient, the average volumetric wear was 30 mm^3 per million

cycles.[13] Therefore, the variable wear rate between patients correlates mostly with the difference in activity levels, and possibly weight, which may explain the difference in survival of total joint implants.

One group studied the wear rates between a highly active group of primary THA patients (alpine and/or cross-country skiing) and a less active group (no winter sports), at 5- and 10-years follow-up. At 5 years, there was a statistically significant higher radiologic sign of loosening in the less active group. However, at 10 years, the more active group showed a higher rate of wear that was statistically significant.[14]

Loading of Total Knee Arthroplasty with General Activities and Sports
D'Lima and colleagues studied in vivo joint loading in TKA patients using a force-sensing device implanted in a custom made tibial component. The implant contained strain gauges to measure three orthogonal and three moment forces acting on the tibial tray. Peak total force was 2.3 × body weight (BW) during walking, 2.5 × BW during chair rise, 3.0 × BW during stair climbing, and 2.1 × BW during squatting.[15] In their study, axial forces predominated, especially in the standing phase of walking; however, overall shear forces, and moments at the tibial tray, were fairly low. The limitations of this study included that it involved only one patient and it was done 3 months postoperative, whereas tibial forces were found to increase up to 2 years postoperatively as shown by the same authors in a later study.[16]

Using the same analysis method as the one used for general activities, the same author published another article concerning sports activities.[17] According to their study, a stationary bicycle produced the lowest load on the knee prosthesis (1.03 ± 0.2 × BW), followed by treadmill walking and elliptical trainer, which had similar knee loads. Other sports are classified from least to most load on the knee joints as follows: gym exercises (leg press, squats, and knee extension), power walking, golf swing (leading knee mostly), tennis, and jogging, which produced forces 4 × BW. A golf swing surprisingly produced a load force on the knee almost as intense as jogging; however, the number of cycles during jogging surpasses by far the number of cycles during a golf game. This explains why most surgeons do not consider golf as a high intensity, whereas they consider jogging as such. Other studies have shown TKA loads of 7 × BW[18] in jogging and even 22 × BW[19] depending on running speed.

One literature review listed TKA joint loading in a wide range of activities (Table 1).[20] Walking loads varied depending on speed (2.8 × BW up to 4.3 × BW). This was also noted in jogging and running, which recorded the highest knee joint load of up to 14 × BW depending on speed. There was a remarkable difference between recreational and skilled skiers (10 and 3.5 × BW, respectively) and different styles (long/short turns, small/large moguls, cross-country classical vs skate skiing) with the former variations having a lower joint load than the latter. For example, small moguls require less joint loads than large moguls.

Loading of Total Hip Arthroplasty with General Activities and Sports

Bergmann and colleagues[21] studied THA loading with general activities in vivo using telemetric data transmission from the used implants. Their study showed that walking (2.34 × BW)

generated less joint loading than standing on one leg. In addition, going downstairs (2.6 × BW) generated more joint loading than going upstairs (2.5 × BW). All other common activities (fast walking, standing up, sitting down) had comparably small joint loading values.

One review of the literature conducted on joint loading of THA (Table 2),[20] found similar loads for activities, such as walking, jogging, cycling, and going up and down the stairs.

PATIENT EXPECTATIONS OF ACTIVITIES

After months of suffering and limitation of activity, patients refer to TJR as a mean of relief and return to an active lifestyle. According to multiple surveys and articles, patients expected pain relief, functional improvement, return to physical activity, and improvement of quality of life.

Meneghini and colleagues[22] used a questionnaire to gather information concerning the

Table 1
Knee joint loading during different activities

Activity	Knee Joint Load (×BW)
Walking at 5.4 km/h	3.4–4
Walking	3.0
Walking at 5 km/h	2.8
Walking at 7 km/h	4.3
Walking	3.5
Cycling at 120 W	1.2
Stair ascent	4.3
Stair ascent	5.0
Stair descent	3.8
Stair descent	6
Ramp ascent	4.5
Ramp descent	4.5
Ramp descent at 5.4 km/h	7–8.5
Squat descent	5.6
Isokinetic knee extension	Up to 9
Jogging at 9 km/h	8–9
Jogging at 12.6 km/h	10.3
Running at 16 km/h	Up to 14
Bowling on asphalt alleys	Up to 12
Skiing medium steep slope	
Beginner	10
Skilled skier	3.5

Courtesy of Kuster M. Exercise Recommendations After Total Joint Replacement. A Review of the Current Literature and Proposal of Scientifically Based Guidelines. Sports Medicine 2002; 32 (7): 433-445.

Table 2
Hip joint loading during different activities

Activity	Hip Joint Load (×BW)
Standing on 2 legs	0.8
Standing on 1 leg	3.2
Straight log raise	1.9
Walking at 1 km/h	2.9
Walking at 5 km/h	4.7
Jogging at 5 km/h	5.0
Jogging at 7 km/h	5.4
Stumbling	8.7
Cycling low resistance (40 W)	0.5
Cycling high resistance	1.4
Jogging at 12 km/h	6
Alpine skiing long turns, flat slope	4.5
Alpine skiing long turns, steep slope	6
Alpine skiing short turns, flat slope	5.5–6
Alpine skiing short turns, steep slope	7–8
Alpine skiing small moguls	8–9
Alpine skiing large moguls	10–15
Cross-country skiing classical	4–5
Cross-country skiing skating	4.5
Walking at natural speed	3.2–6.2
Stair ascent	3.4–6
Car entry	5–8
Car exit	4.5–8
Bath entry	4.6–6.6
Stair ascent	5
Stair descent	5.6
Ramp ascent	6.8
Ramp descent	6.5

Courtesy of Kuster M. Exercise Recommendations After Total Joint Replacement. A Review of the Current Literature and Proposal of Scientifically Based Guidelines. Sports Medicine 2002; 32 (7): 433-445.

expectations of patients and their knowledge on TKA. Their study showed that 81% of patients expected the surgery to alleviate their pain, whereas 19% wanted mostly to return to sport activities. Furthermore, 37% expected that TKA would last more than 20 years, and that was because of their exposure to traditional news media and to the Internet. It has been shown that patients may have unrealistically high expectations for total knee replacement, which can be caused by their constant exposure to media and Internet.[23,24]

Another study showed that at 5-year follow-up post-TKA, expectations for physical activity were higher than their actual ability to perform postoperatively.[25] It concluded that most patient were able to achieve the desired pain control; however, their expectations of physical activity were not fulfilled to the same extent.

On another note, one-quarter of patients with osteoarthritis claim that it limited their sexual activity (SA) and contributed to marital unhappiness.[26,27] According to Harmsen and colleagues,[28] 63% of patients expected to resume SA after THA. Unfortunately, 43% of these patients were unsatisfied with the outcome at 1-year follow-up, highlighting the complex reasons for reduction of SA in relationships. However, one-fifth of those who did not expect it were sexually active within the same time period. Accordingly, the authors recommended that clinicians inform patients (elderly in particular) to have realistic expectations regarding SA post-THA.

A large survey that included 20 hospitals in the Netherlands was conducted to ask patients about their expectations from undergoing TJR (52% were THA patients).[29] The most common reason for surgery was improvement of function (43%) followed by pain relief (35%). In their survey, patient who could not choose between pain relief and improvement of function as their expectation showed more improvement in outcomes compared with patients who could. In addition, patients who expected pain relief were clinically worse before surgery than patients who expected improvement in function and were more satisfied with the outcome. As a result, they proved that patient's expectations can predict to a certain extent the satisfaction level with a desired outcome. As such it is of critical importance for physicians to discuss these expectations in advance with their patients, because patient expectations may not be realistic. Unfulfilled expectations are the principal source of dissatisfaction after joint replacement, especially after TKR.[30,31]

PHYSICIAN RECOMMENDATIONS FOR ACTIVITY

In 1999, researchers conducted a survey on members of the Hip Society.[32] They recommended 10 low-impact activities (including golf, speed walking, and road cycling), recommended with experience seven moderate-impact activities (including downhill skiing and weight lifting), and did not recommend 10 high-impact activities (eg, jogging, contact sports, and snowboarding). It was curious why skiing was considered acceptable and snowboarding was not, and it is perhaps a reflection of the age group of the respondents who would have been more knowledgeable about skiing than snowboarding because in 1999 snowboarding would have been a sport of younger individuals.

At the 2007 annual meeting of the American Association for Hip and Knee Surgeons (AAHKS), a large survey was performed to review physician recommendations for activity post-THA and TKA surgeries (Fig. 1).[6] There was a general consensus concerning placing no limitation on walking and cycling on even surfaces, swimming, climbing stairs, and golf and discouraging high-impact activities, such as sprinting, jogging, and skiing on difficult terrain for THA and TKA. However, a significant difference was noted in intermediate-impact activities, such as tennis, off-road cycling, and skiing on groomed trails. In addition, surgeon recommendations were more lenient toward THA patients than TKA patients (statistically significant) in regards to singles and doubles tennis, walking uphill, and jogging.

Trying to compare the evolution of physician recommendations over the years, Healy and colleagues compared the results of surveys completed by members of the Hip Society and Knee Society between 1999 and 2005 (**Tables 3** and **4**).[33] During this 6-year period, joint replacement experts decreased their restrictions on sports and allowed their patients more physical activities. Therefore, the trend is to give patients more freedom in choosing the lifestyle and physical activities that suits them best. Although this is not an evidence-based evolution, several factors have influenced expert recommendations including higher patient demands, rising confidence in surgical techniques, biomaterial advancement, and innovations in joint implants.

ACTUAL PATIENT'S POSTOPERATIVE ACTIVITIES

According to multiple studies, 10,000 steps per day are recommended to achieve and maintain the health benefits of physical activity.[34–36] A meta-analysis included 20 studies using accelerometers and pedometers to assess the physical activity of post-TJR patients.[37] On average, TJR patients performed 6721 steps per day. A meta-regression showed that walking activity decreased by 90 steps per day every year after surgery.

It seems that TJR patients are less active than what is recommended to maintain a healthy lifestyle. However, it has been shown that these numbers vary significantly with age. Bohannon[38] showed in his meta-analysis that healthy people older than 65 years take 6565 steps per day, whereas those younger than 65 years take 9800 steps per day.

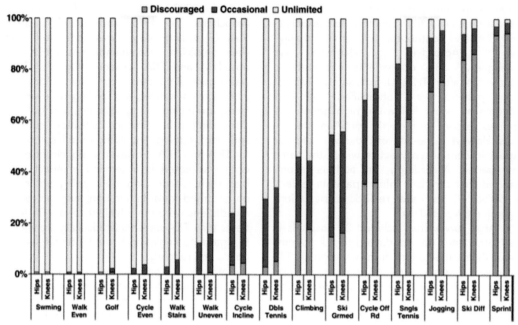

Fig. 1. Graph of physician activity recommendations after THA and TKA. Survey by the AAHKS. (*Courtesy of* Swanson EA, Schmalzried TP, Dorey FJ. Activity recommendations after total hip and knee arthroplasty: a survey of the American Association for Hip and Knee Surgeons. The Journal of Arthroplasty Vol. 24 No. 6 Suppl. 1 2009 (https://doi.org/10.1016/j.arth.2009.05.014).)

On another note, a survey[39] showed that 44% of patients who were engaged in sports before surgery resumed it post-THA. In addition, 71% of these patients reported to have an equal or better athletic performance than before surgery. However, there was a statistically significant difference in body mass index (BMI) between patients who did and those who did not return to sports (RTS). Among those who did not resume sports, 50% were overweight or obese. When asked about the reason for not resuming sports, the most common answer was fear of damaging the prosthesis, followed by pain and surgeon's recommendations.

Using a cross-sectional survey in a tertiary care arthroplasty center, involving primary THA and TKA patients, one study[40] found that the median University of California Los Angeles (UCLA) activity score was 6 (scale of 1–9) corresponding to a moderate level of activity. The mean follow-up was 40.7 months for hips and 36.6 months for knees. In addition, at 1-year follow-up, the mean Harris Hip Score was 94.8, Oxford Hip Score was 16.6, Knee Society Score clinical score was 95.9, Knee Society Score function score was 95.0, and Oxford Knee Score was 18.2. Accordingly, TJR patients are able to undergo an active lifestyle with mild to moderate level of activity.

RETURN TO WORK FOLLOWING TOTAL JOINT REPLACEMENT

The working population constitutes a substantial portion of TJR patients. According to the National Registry of England and Wales, 40% of THA and 32% of TKA patients were less than 65 years of age at the time of surgery.[41] McGonagle and colleagues[42] showed a return to work (RTW) rate of 91% after a mean of 6.4 weeks for THA patients and 7.7 weeks for TKA patients. In this survey, there was a nonsignificant correlation between time to RTW and physical demands of the work (P = .28), or with the type of surgery (P = .18). However, when working hours were flexible, it significantly decreased the time to RTW (P = .03). Other favorable factors for earlier RTW were active recovery, proper physiotherapy, psychological factors (desire, boredom), and financial necessity.

The ability to drive has a large impact on patient independence, RTW, and ability to fulfill the requirements of daily living. According to Rondon and colleagues,[43] on average, patients returned to driving at 4.4 and 3.7 weeks for TKA and THA (P = .001), respectively. Surprisingly, right-sided procedures only added an average of 1.7 and 1.6 days for TKA and THA,

Table 3
Comparison of results of the Hip Society surveys in 1999 and 2005

Allowed			Allowed with Experience			No Consensus			Not Recommended		
	1999	2005		1999	2005		1999	2005		1999	2005
Stationary cycling	✓	✓	Bowling	✓		Square dancing	✓		Baseball	✓	
Ballroom dancing	✓	✓	Canoeing	✓		Fencing	✓	✓	Basketball	✓	✓
Golf	✓	✓	Road cycling	✓		Rowing	✓		Football	✓	✓
Shuffleboard	✓	✓	Hiking	✓		Ice skating	✓		Gymnastics	✓	
Swimming	✓	✓	Horseback riding	✓	✓	Roller skating	✓		Handball	✓	
Doubles tennis	✓	✓	Cross-country skiing	✓	✓	Downhill skiing	✓		Hockey	✓	✓
Normal walking	✓	✓	Rowing		✓	Stationary skiing	✓		Jogging	✓	
Bowling		✓	Ice skating		✓	Speed walking	✓		Rock climbing	✓	
Canoeing		✓	Roller skating		✓	Weight lifting	✓		Soccer	✓	✓
Road cycling		✓	Downhill skiing		✓	Weight machine	✓		Squash/racquetball	✓	
Square dancing		✓	Stationary skiing		✓	Baseball		✓	Singles tennis	✓	
Hiking		✓	Doubles tennis		✓	Gymnastics		✓	Volleyball	✓	

(continued on next page)

Activity	Allowed		Allowed with Experience		No Consensus		Not Recommended	
	1999	2005	1999	2005	1999	2005	1999	2005
Speed walking		✓						
Weight lifting				✓				
Weight machine				✓				
Handball						✓		
Hockey						✓		
Rock climbing						✓		
Squash/racquetball						✓		
Singles tennis						✓		
Volleyball						✓		

Courtesy of Healy WL, Sharma S, Schwartz B, Iorio R. Current Concepts Review: Athletic Activity After Total Joint Arthroplasty. JBJS VOLUME 90-A. NUMBER 10. OCTOBER 2008 (2008;90:2245-52).

Table 4
Comparison of results of the Knee Society surveys in 1999 and 2005

Allowed

Activity	1999	2005
Bowling	✓	✓
Stationary cycling	✓	✓
Ballroom dancing	✓	✓
Golf	✓	✓
Horseback riding	✓	✓
Shuffleboard	✓	✓
Swimming	✓	✓
Normal walking	✓	✓
Canoeing		✓
Road cycling		✓
Square dancing		✓
Hiking		✓
Speed walking		✓

Allowed with Experience

Activity	1999	2005
Canoeing	✓	
Road cycling	✓	
Hiking	✓	
Rowing	✓	✓
Ice skating	✓	✓
Cross-country skiing	✓	✓
Stationary skiing	✓	✓
Doubles tennis	✓	✓
Speed walking	✓	
Weight machine	✓	✓
Horseback riding		✓
Downhill skiing		✓

No Consensus

Activity	1999	2005
Square dancing	✓	
Fencing	✓	✓
Roller skating	✓	✓
Downhill skiing	✓	
Weight lifting	✓	✓
Baseball		✓
Gymnastics		✓
Handball		✓
Hockey		✓
Rock climbing		✓
Squash/racquetball		✓
Singles tennis		✓
Weight machine		

Not Recommended

Activity	1999	2005
Baseball	✓	
Basketball	✓	✓
Football	✓	✓
Gymnastics	✓	
Handball	✓	
Hockey	✓	
Jogging	✓	✓
Rock climbing	✓	
Soccer	✓	✓
Squash/racquetball	✓	
Singles tennis	✓	
Volleyball	✓	✓

Courtesy of Healy WL, Sharma S, Schwartz B, Iorio R. Current Concepts Review: Athletic Activity After Total Joint Arthroplasty. JBJS VOLUME 90-A. NUMBER 10. OCTOBER 2008 (2008;90:2245-52).

respectively. Most patients returned to driving within 12 weeks of surgery.

A recent meta-analysis examined total brake response time (TBRT) as an indicator for safe return to driving. It concluded that right-sided THA and right-sided TKA returned to baseline TBRT at 2 and 4 weeks after surgery, respectively.[44] In addition, laterality has a significant influence on return to drive timing. A systematic review found that patients returned to TBRT within 1 week following left-sided procedures compared with 4 weeks following right-sided procedures.[45]

On a larger scale, a systematic review[46] was conducted with 19 articles published between 1984 and 2013 with a total of 4521 TJR patients. The proportions of patients returning to work ranged from 25% to 95% at 1 to 12 months after THA and from 71% to 83% at 3 to 6 months after TKA. RTW after THA ranged from 1.1 to 10.5 weeks and after TKA ranged from 8 to 12 weeks.

Overall most studies show that most of the previously working patients returned to work after TJR, with THA patients returning earlier than TKA patients and work status affected by sociodemographic, health, and job characteristics.

RETURN TO SPORTS FOLLOWING TOTAL JOINT REPLACEMENT

With the evolution of joint-replacement surgery and its adaptation to a younger population, the expected goals and outcomes from these operations is no longer confined to pain management and better quality of life. Patient expectations grew larger to include a more active life and return to their previous sports levels.

A large systematic review[47] of 42 papers that included a total of 10,758 with average age of 61.7, showed an RTS rate between 54% and 98%. Younger age, lower BMI, sports practice preoperatively, absence of other joint pain, and males were associated with higher levels of activity. No significant difference in performance was noted between THA and TKA patients; however, in one study THA patients had a better rate of RTS.[48] Furthermore, none of the studies showed an increase in complication rates with sporting activity with respect to the less-active control subjects. Some studies showed an increase in wear rates in the more active groups but without an increase in revision rates.[49,50]

Timing of RTS is controversial. Multiple confounding variables affect the ability to judge the ideal time for a TJR patient to resume his or her sporting activities. A recent meta-analysis showed an average time of 13 weeks after TKA to RTS, of which 95% concerned low-impact sports.

Thirty-three percent of AAHKS members recommended their patients to return to allowable (as per their guidelines) sports within the first 3 months postoperatively compared with 24% from the Hip Society; however, these differences were not statistically significant. However, recommendations for RTS at 3 to 6 months were significant. Seventy-one percent of the Hip Society members and 58.4% of AAHKS recommended this time period.[51] The senior author does not impose a time limit as to when patients RTS. Patients are allowed to return to any activity whenever they believe that they are physically capable of doing it.

FACTORS INFLUENCING RETURN TO ACTIVITY

Patients undergoing TJR are subject to multiple factors influencing their ability to return to their previous level of activity. According to a large systematic review that included 19 studies,[46] factors associated with worse RTW outcomes included female gender, older age, pain in joints other than the hips, surgical complication, physical work, unskilled work, and being a farmer. In addition, younger age, working until 1 month preoperatively, primary arthritis, higher education level, and having a better postoperative walking ability were associated with better outcomes. Preoperative function, type of prosthesis, and surgical procedure did not significantly affect the postoperative work status.

Using the UCLA score at 1-year post-TJR, a large retrospective study showed that preoperative UCLA activity score, age, male sex, and BMI were predictors of higher sports activity level, whereas the type of surgery and implant characteristics did not.[52]

Bradbury and colleagues[53] found that medical comorbidities and perioperative complications negatively influenced RTS, whereas motivation and preoperative sports level had a positive effect. Discouragement from their surgeons, mainly to high-impact types of sports, was mentioned as a negative confounder of RTS in multiple studies.[48]

SUMMARY

Activity level after TJR and influencing factors, prosthetic loading and wear, timing and ability to RTW or sports, and physician recommendations are all controversial topics addressed in this review. In general, most TJR patients are able to return to their previous level of activity and to a lesser extent to sports. Despite guidelines being set by large expert societies, final recommendations should be individualized and based on patient characteristics, realistic expectations, and medical status. Finally, the literature is sparse on long-term outcomes of high-level activity on implant durability and survival. We recommend intensifying research regarding this subject to be able to find more solid recommendations, especially regarding high-impact sports and athletic activities.

CLINICS CARE POINTS

- TJR patients are increasingly seeking a more active lifestyle, trying to return to their previous levels of activity.
- Wear is a function of use.
- Patient preoperative expectations dictates postoperative satisfaction.
- Experts recommendations of activity for TJR patients are becoming more and more lenient.
- Most TJR patients are able to RTW and RTS with several confounding variables including age, BMI, preoperative level of activity, and medical comorbidities.
- No solid evidence on long-term effect of high level of activity on implants survival.

DISCLOSURE

Institutional Support by Smith and Nephew, Styker, DePuy and Zimmer.

REFERENCES

1. Lee IM, Skerrett PJ. Physical activity and all-cause mortality: what is the dose-response relation? Med Sci Sports Exerc 2001;33(suppl):S459–71 [discussion: S493–4].
2. Macera CA, Ham SA, Yore MM, et al. Prevalence of physical activity in the United States: behavioral risk factor surveillance system, 2001. Prev Chronic Dis 2005;2:A17.
3. American College of Sports Medicine Physicians Statement. The recommended quantity and quality of exercise for developing and maintaining cardiovascular and muscular fitness in healthy adults. Med Sci Sports Exerc 1990;22(2):265–74.
4. Perruccio AV, Bradley EM, Guan J. Burden of disease. In: Bradley EM, Glazier RH, editors. Arthritis and related conditions in Ontario: ICES research atlas. 2nd edition. Toronto (Canada): Institute for Clinical Evaluative Sciences; 2004;2:15-40.
5. Sloan M, Premkumar A, Sheth NP. Projected volume of primary total joint arthroplasty in the U.S., 2014 to 2030. J Bone Joint Surg Am 2018;100(17): 1455–60.
6. Swanson EA, Schmalzried TP, Dorey FJ. Activity recommendations after total hip and knee arthroplasty: a survey of the American Association for Hip and Knee Surgeons. J Arthroplasty 2009;24(6 suppl):120–6.
7. Schmalzried TP, Callaghan JJ. Wear in total hip and knee replacements. J Bone Joint Surg Am 1999; 81(1):115–36.
8. Horikoshi M, Macaulay W, Booth RE, et al. Comparison of interface membranes obtained from failed cemented and cementless hip and knee prostheses. Clin Orthop 1994;(309):69–87.
9. Kuster MS, Stachowiak GW. Factors affecting polyethylene wear in total knee replacement. Orthopedics 2002;25(2 Suppl):S235–42.
10. Stern SH, Bowen MK, Insall JN, et al. Cemented total knee arthroplasty for gonarthrosis in patients 55 years old or younger. Clin Orthop 1990;(260):124–919.
11. Diduch DR, Insall JN, Scott WN, et al. Total knee replacement in young, active patients: long-term follow-up and functional outcome. J Bone Joint Surg Am 1997;79(4):575–82.
12. Schmalzried TP, Szuszczewicz ES, NorthfieldMR, et al. Quantitative assessment of walking activity after total hip or knee replacement. J Bone Joint Surg Am 1998;80(1):54–9.
13. Schmalzried TP, Shepherd EF, Dorey FJ, et al. The John Charnley Award: wear is a function of use, not time. Clin Orthop 2000;(381):36–46.
14. Gschwend N, Frei T, Morscher E, et al. Alpine and cross-country skiing after total hip replacement. Acta Orthop Scand 2000;71(3):243–9.
15. Darryl D, D'Lima B, Patila S, et al. In vivo knee moments and shear after total knee arthroplasty. J Biomech 2007;40:S11–7.
16. D'Lima DD, Patil S, Steklov N, et al. The Chitranjan Ranawat Award: in vivo knee forces after total knee arthroplasty. Clin Orthop Relat Res 2005;440:45–9.
17. D'Lima DD, Steklov N, Patil S, et al. In vivo knee forces during recreation and exercise after knee arthroplasty. Clin Orthop Relat Res 2008;466: 2605–11.
18. Glitsch U, Baumann W. The three-dimensional determination of internal loads in the lower extremity. J Biomech 1997;30:1123–31.
19. Harrison RN, Lees A, McCullagh PJ, et al. A bioengineering analysis of human muscle and joint forces in the lower limbs during running. J Sports Sci 1986;4(3):201–18.
20. Kuster M. Exercise recommendations after total joint replacement. a review of the current literature and proposal of scientifically based guidelines. Sports Med 2002;32(7):433–45.

21. Bergmann G, Deuretzbacher G, Heller M, et al. Hip contact forces and gait patterns from routine activities. J Biomech 2001;34(7):859–71.

22. Meneghini RM, Russo GS, Lieberman JR. Modern perceptions and expectations regarding total knee arthroplasty. J Knee Surg 2014;27:93–8.

23. Hepinstall MS, Rutledge JR, Bornstein LJ, et al. Factors that impact expectations before total knee arthroplasty. J Arthroplasty 2011;26(6):870–6.

24. Mannion AF, Kämpfen S, Munzinger U, et al. The role of patient expectations in predicting outcome after total knee arthroplasty. Arthritis Res Ther 2009;11(5):R139.

25. Nilsdotter AK, Toksvig-Larsen S, Roos EM. Knee arthroplasty: are patients' expectations fulfilled? A prospective study of pain and function in 102 patients with 5-year follow-up. Acta Orthop 2009; 80(1):55–61.

26. Laffosse JM, Tricoire JL, Chiron P, et al. Sexual function before and after primary total hip arthroplasty. Joint Bone Spine 2008;75(2):189–94.

27. Meyer H, Stern R, Fusetti C, et al. Sexual quality of life after hip surgery. J Orthop Traumatol 2003;4(1):21–5.

28. Harmsen RT, Den Oudsten BL, Putter H, et al. Patient expectations of sexual activity after total hip arthroplasty. JB JS Open Access 2018;3:e0031.

29. Wiering B, de Boer D, Delnoij D. Meeting patient expectations: patient expectations and recovery after hip or knee surgery. Musculoskelet Surg 2018; 102:231–40.

30. Bourne RB, Chesworth BM, Davis AM, et al. Patient satisfaction after total knee arthroplasty: who is satisfied and who is not? Clin Orthop Relat Res 2010;468(1):57–63.

31. Noble PC, Conditt MA, Cook KF, et al. The John Insall Award: patient expectations affect satisfaction with total knee arthroplasty. Clin Orthop Relat Res 2006;452:35–43.

32. Healy WL, Iorio R, Lemos MJ. Athletic activity after joint replacement. Am J Sports Med 2001;29: 377–88.

33. Healy WL, Sharma S, Schwartz B, et al. Current concepts review: athletic activity after total joint arthroplasty. J Bone Joint Surg Am 2008;90(10):2245–52.

34. Iwane M, Arita M, Tomimoto S, et al. Walking 10,000 steps/day or more reduces blood pressure and sympathetic nerve activity in mild essential hypertension. Hypertens Res 2000;23:573–80.

35. Tudor-Locke C, Hatano Y, Pangrazi RP, et al. Revisiting 'how many steps are enough? Med Sci Sports Exerc 2008;40(suppl):S537–43.

36. Schneider PL, Bassett DR Jr, Thompson DL, et al. Effects of a 10,000 steps per day goal in overweight adults. Am J Health Promot 2006;21:85–9.

37. Naal FD, Impellizzeri FM. How active are patients undergoing total joint arthroplasty? A systematic review. Clin Orthop Relat Res 2010;468:1891–904.

38. Bohannon RW. Number of pedometer-assessed steps taken per day by adults: a descriptive meta-analysis. Phys Ther 2007;87:1642–50.

39. Madrid J, Bautista M, Guio JF, et al. Perceived skills for sports performance after primary hip arthroplasty: a cross-sectional study. Int Orthopaedics 2019;43:2725–30.

40. Bauman S, Williams D, Petruccelli D, et al. Physical activity after total joint replacement: a cross-sectional survey. Clin J Sport Med 2007;17:104–8.

41. The NJR Editorial Board (2016) National Joint Registry for England, Wales, Northern Ireland and the Isle of Man. In: 14th Annual Report of the National Joint Registry for England, Wales, Northern Ireland and the Isle of Man, 2016.

42. McGonagle L, Convery-Chan L, DeCruz P, et al. Factors influencing return to work after hip and knee arthroplasty. J Orthop Traumatol 2019;20:9.

43. Rondon AJ, Tan TL, Goswami K, et al. When can I drive? Predictors of returning to driving after total joint arthroplasty. J Am Acad Orthop Surg 2019;00:1–7.

44. van der Velden CA, Tolk JJ, Janssen RPA, et al. When is it safe to resume driving after total hip and total knee arthroplasty? A meta-analysis of literature on post-operative brake reaction times. Bone Joint J 2017;99-B:566–76.

45. DiSilvestro KJ, Santoro AJ, Tjoumakaris FP, et al. When can I drive after orthopaedic surgery? A systematic review. Clin Orthop Relat Res 2016;474: 2557–70.

46. Tilbury C, Schaasberg W, Plevier JW, et al. Return to work after total hip and knee arthroplasty: a systematic review. Rheumatology (Oxford) 2014;53(3):512–25.

47. Jassim SS, Douglas SL, Haddad FS. Athletic activity after lower limb arthroplasty: a systematic review of current evidence. Bone Joint J 2014;96-B:923–7.

48. Huch K, Müller KA, Stürmer T, et al. Sports activities 5 years after total knee or hip arthroplasty: the Ulm Osteoarthritis Study. Ann Rheum Dis 2005;64:1715–20.

49. Lavernia CJ, Sierra RJ, Hungerford DS, et al. Activity level and wear in total knee arthroplasty: a study of autopsy retrieved specimens. J Arthroplasty 2001;16:446–53.

50. Ollivier M, Frey S, Parratte S, et al. Does impact sport activity influence total hip arthroplasty durability? Clin Orthop Relat Res 2012;470:3060–6.

51. Klein GR, Levine BR, Hozack WJ, et al. Return to athletic activity after total hip arthroplasty. consensus guidelines based on a survey of the hip Society and American Association of Hip and Knee Surgeons. J Arthroplasty 2007;22(2):171–5.

52. Williams DH, Greidanus NV, Masri BA, et al. Predictors of participation in sports after hip and knee arthroplasty. Clin Orthop Relat Res 2012;470:555–61.

53. Bradbury N, Borton D, Spoo G, et al. Participation in sports after total knee replacement. Am J Sports Med 1998;26(4):530–5.

Does Multimodal Therapy Influence Functional Outcome After Total Knee Arthroplasty?

Ahmed A. Magan, BM, BSc, MRCS, FRCS(Tr & Orth)[a],[*],
Syed S. Ahmed, MBChB, LLM, MSc, FRCS (Tr & Orth)[a],
Bruce Paton, BAppSc, PhD[a],[b],
Sujith Konan, MBBS, MD (Res), MRCS, FRCS(Tr &Orth)[a],
Fares S. Haddad, BSc, MD (Res), MCh(Orth), FRCS(Orth), FFSEM[a],[b],[c]

KEYWORDS

- Psychometrics • Outcome of total knee arthroplasty • Multimodal therapy in OA • SF-12
- Level of evidence level II

KEY POINTS

- Psychosocial health plays an important role in patients diagnosed with osteoarthritis of the knee.
- Multimodal therapy improves patient-reported outcomes in patients who are treated non-operatively or operatively.
- Importantly, multimodal therapy classes have a positive impact on the mental subscale of SF12 scores following primary TKA.

INTRODUCTION

The 16th National Joint Registry (NJR) for England, Wales, and Northern Ireland reported that 102,944 primary knee replacements were undertaken from 2018 to 2019 of which 90,089 were total knee arthroplasty (TKA).[1] As expected, there was a slight increase in the incidence of revision TKAs. The approximate revision rate over 15 years is now at 4.47% according to the latest NJR report. Furthermore, pooled survival data from the various registries show survivorship at 15 years to be around 93%.[2]

The patient-reported outcome measures (PROMs) after primary TKAs have shown an overall improvement in recent years. However, the proportion of patients who were satisfied with the outcomes is lower than the ratings for hip surgery on the same items of PROMs. Studies have highlighted this concern regarding variations in functional outcome and rate of recovery after TKA. Up to 20% of patients are not entirely satisfied with their outcome.[3]

One in 8 patients may have persistent pain postoperatively despite well-fitting and functioning implants.[4] The cause for this dissatisfaction is multifactorial. Rarely do physicians find a significant cause such as mechanical malalignment, loosening, or infection. Some studies have also documented a deterioration in function after TKA surgery; for example, 1 study found that 11% of patients thought function was the same or worse than it was preoperatively at a minimum of 2 years following surgery.[5]

Several studies have tried to ascertain factors that influence outcome and satisfaction

[a] Univerisity College London Hospital NHS Foundation Trust, London, UK; [b] The Institute of Sports, Exercise and Health, London, UK; [c] The Princess Grace Hospital, London, UK
* Corresponding author.
E-mail address: ahmedmagan@gmail.com

Orthop Clin N Am 51 (2020) 453–459
https://doi.org/10.1016/j.ocl.2020.06.011

following TKA.[5–9] It has been shown that preoperative pain and physical function are the strongest predictors of postoperative pain and physical function.[10,11] However, these alone do not explain the high variability in postoperative outcomes and recovery. There has been an increased interest in the influence of psychosocial health on the outcomes after knee arthroplasty.[3,12]

The National Health Service in the United Kingdom links reimbursement to patient outcomes. Similar scenarios are seen in Canada and the United States. Therefore, it is critical to understand better the factors that influence patient outcome after primary TKA. More importantly, it is crucial to identify interventions that would positively influence patients' perception of surgical outcomes and improve psychosocial health, such that it could be harnessed to improve overall functional outcome.

A previous study from the authors' institution revealed that in cases amenable to nonoperative treatment, a multimodal intervention encompassing education, diet, and physiotherapy has an excellent impact on improving the symptoms of mild-to-moderate osteoarthritis of the knee at 1 year.[13]

The authors hypothesized that if psychosocial health has an influence on outcomes after TKA, an intervention addressing psychosocial health such as education, exercises, and counseling will certainly have an effect on the outcomes (eg, pain, function, and satisfaction) measured after primary TKA.

Study questions were

> Does multimodal therapy influence the quality of life and function in patients diagnosed with osteoarthritis of the knee joint?
> In patients who proceed to have a TKA after multimodal therapy, can the response to the multimodal therapy influence the overall functional outcome of surgery?

METHODS
Study Design and Setting
Patients diagnosed with osteoarthritis of the knee were enrolled in the study and prospectively followed. All patients had symptomatic knee osteoarthritis and were registered in the lower limb classes at a large teaching hospital. All patients who had osteoarthritis were included in the study. Only patients not willing to attend classes were excluded from the study.

Participants/Study Subjects
Five hundred twenty-six patients (181 male, 345 female) were enrolled and available for the study. Forty-five patients did not consent or failed to attend classes and were excluded. The mean follow-up was 48 months (4–72 months). Of these, 133 patients (41 male, 72 female) underwent TKA.

DESCRIPTION OF EXPERIMENT, TREATMENT, OR SURGERY
Multimodal Lower Limb Classes
All participants were enrolled for 12 classes lasting 60 minutes over 6 weeks (Box 1). Apart from an exercise program, the class also included physiotherapist-led education and a weight management lecture by a dietitian. Patients were educated on safety, disease pathology and progression, the effect of exercise on joints, footwear, and orthotics. They were also informed on how to minimize complications such as swelling and pain following each class. The exercise program was part of each class and targeted joint flexibility, muscle strength, cardiovascular training, balance, and proprioception. This involved stretching and warm-up exercises for 15 minutes followed by 10 circuit stations.

Each circuit station lasted 1 minute initially, with 2 minutes recovery time between stations. The station time was progressively increased to 3 minutes, with a 1 minute recovery station in the final week of the program. Written information was given at the end of the last class on local community-run exercise program, which enabled patients to manage their exercises and activities.

VARIABLES, OUTCOME MEASURES, AND DATA SOURCES

Following informed consent, patients were prospectively followed for up to 72 months. All patients were asked to complete questionnaires to evaluate their Oxford knee score (OKS), pain scores (visual analogue score [VAS]), SF12 Score and Western Ontario and McMaster Universities Osteoarthritis Index (WOMAC) pain, stiffness, and physical function subscales to obtain baseline values. With respect to the WOMAC subscales, these values were added to give a cumulative WOMAC score. Patients were longitudinally followed to determine whether there was a change in these scores. Follow-up questionnaires were collected at the time of recruitment, at 6 weeks, 3 months, 6 months, 12 months and then annually. In patients

Box 1
Total knee arthroplasty multimodal therapy program

1. Six-week program
   a. 2 x 1-h sessions per week
2. Circuit group participants
   a. 10 × 30 s stations (increased by 30s/station/wk) and consisting of;
      i. Warm-up for 15 minutes
      ii. Range of movement and flexibility work
      iii. Leg press
      iv. Stationary bike interval work-cardiovascular fitness
      v. Functional exercises-sit to stand and steps.
      vi. Exercising glutes, hamstring, and calf muscles.
      vii. Proprioceptive and balance work.
3. Postclass education on the following
   a. Surgery and recovery plans
   b. Rehabilitation goals
   c. Dietician (focusing on weight management)
   d. Pain management
   e. Maintaining exercise and physical activity before and after surgery
   f. Removing barriers to ongoing exercise maintenance
4. Relevant outcome scores collected
   a. WOMAC
   b. SF12
   c. OKS

outcome measure. It has straightforward scoring methodology that makes it an excellent choice for the evaluation of patients with hip and knee osteoarthritis. This score has undergone rigorous validations and consists of 24 questions in 3 domains of pain, stiffness, and physical function. Each answer is scored on a scale of 0 to 4, with a lower score reflecting fewer symptoms or disability.

The SF-12 consists of 12 items that assess 8 dimensions of health: physical functioning, role-physical, bodily pain, general health, vitality, social functioning, role emotional, and mental health. The SF-12 a score for 0 to 100, with the highest score indicating best health.

The OKS is a 12-item patient-reported PROM specifically designed and developed to assess function and pain after TKA. It is short, reproducible, valid and sensitive to clinically significant changes. It is a simple scoring system that eliminates interobserver error as it is completed by the patient independent of the clinical team. It has a score from 0 to 48, with a maximum score indicating best outcome.

Parametric tests were used for the normally distributed data (Independent T-test and paired T-test) and nonparametric tests for non-normally distributed data (Mann-Whitney test and Wilcoxon Signed Ranks test) to compare the groups for improvement in outcomes after surgery. Effect size (Cohen d) and Pearson correlation were used to document any difference in the improvement of outcome scores between groups that were compared. Regression analysis was used to test the association between change in SF-12 MCS score and the postoperative function scores.

All statistical analyses were done with the use of SPSS (version 13, Chicago, Illinois). A statistical value of $P<.05$ was considered to be significant.

undergoing TKA, postoperative questionnaires were collected at 6 weeks, 3 months, 6 months, 12 months, and then annually.

Statistical Analysis, Study Size

Baseline outcome scores before intervention were used as controls. Statistical difference between the functional outcomes for the control and treated groups was evaluated using a dependent t-test for paired samples.

Functional outcomes, WOMAC scores, OKS, SF-12 physical component subscale (PCS) and pain scores (PS) were compared preoperatively and at the latest follow up postoperatively. The WOMAC score is a popular patient-reported

RESULTS

The multimodal therapy program improved the SF-12, OKS, pain scores (visual analogue scale [VAS]) and WOMAC scores significantly (Table 1).

133 patients (41 male, 72 female) from the total study cohort went on to have TKA at an average of 6 months (range 4–24 months) after multimodal therapy. The indication was clinical deterioration of pain and function. There were 41 males and 72 females patients. The average age was 67 years (range 58–84 years). They all had the same TKA, which included a patellar resurfacing.

Table 1
The multimodal therapy program improved the outcome in the osteoarthritis knee

	SF 12 PCS		SF 12 MCS		WOMAC		OKS		Pain (VAS)	
	Pre	Post	Pre	Post	Pre	Post	Pre	Post	Pre	Post
Average	34.40	35.32	44.62	47.61	65.61	57.94	35.41	32.96	5.91	5.05
Min	14.80	15.00	13.50	17.10	26.00	0.00	0.48	0.52	1.00	1.00
Max	57.10	58.60	68.40	70.10	62.00	62.00	57.00	55.00	10.00	10.00
STDEV	9.08	9.93	11.32	11.54	20.76	23.01	9.79	9.90	2.20	2.19
P value	.04		.009		.001		.013		0	

The postmultimodal SF-12 MCS in this group was identified to segregate this cohort into 2 groups. Group I showed improvement in SF-12 MCS after multimodal therapy. Group II did not show this improvement. Comparison of demographic data between the 2 groups illustrated no significant difference between the groups (Table 2). Subgroup analysis of those patients who had undergone arthroplasty demonstrated that the multimodal classes led toward a nonsignificant deterioration in both WOMAC and OKS before they proceeded to surgical intervention. The mean WOMAC score changed from 65.61 to 57.94. (P=.001) and the mean OKS changed from 35.41 to 32.96 (P = .013, see Table 1). No significant correlation was demonstrated between the number of classes attended and percentage change in outcome measure (Spearman rho 0.012 for WOMAC and 0.017 for OKS).

These 2 subgroups groups were compared for change in postoperative functional and pain scores. After TKA, both groups showed a statistically significant improvement in postoperative WOMAC scores, SF-12 PCS and MCS scores and OKS (Table 3). Patients who showed an improved MCS following multimodal therapy had a greater effect size in their change in WOMAC, OKS, and PCS (see Table 3). Multimodal therapy was associated with a measurable improvement in function pain and health status

at a mean follow-up of 12 months (range 4–24 months).

Regression analysis showed that the change in SF-12 MCS after multimodal therapy strongly predicted the WOMAC score at 12 months, with a range of follow-up of 4 to 24 months (regression coefficient 0.78, [95% confidence interval (CI) 0.34–1.34] standard error 0.19, P=.0001). The change in SF-12 MCS after multimodal therapy moderately predicted the OKS score at 4 to 24 months follow-up (regression coefficient 0.49, [95% CI 0.32–0.51], standard error 0.13, P=.005).

DISCUSSION

This study demonstrates that a multimodal program consisting of nonoperative interventions

Table 2
Demographic data comparing the groups that showed or did not show changes in SF12 MCS

Feature	MCS Improved	MCS Not Improved
Average age (SD) yrs	68 (11)	67 (13)
Male (%)	30.4	31.2
BMI (SD)	30.3 (6.5)	30.4 (6.5)

Table 3
Patients who showed an improved MCS following multimodal therapy had a greater effect size in their change in WOMAC, OKS and MCS

Changes in WOMAC, OKS and SF-12 Scores and Effect Sizes				
SF-12 MCS Score Change	Pre	Post	P-Value	Effect Size [r]
WOMAC				
Improved	58.1	7.8	.02	0.81
Not improved	60.4	12.4	.04	0.13
OKS				
Improved	38.64	12.4	.01	0.79
Not improved	40.1	18.7	.04	0.34
SF-12 MCS				
Improved	34.89	35.41	.02	0.61
Not improved	32.15	36.57	.03	0.21
Pain score (VAS)				
Improved	9.3	3.4	.05	0.56
Not improved	9.6	6.5	.44	0.04

has a positive impact on the symptoms of osteo-arthritis of the knee. Moreover, patients who show improvement in psychosocial health following such intervention have a better functional outcome following TKA. This was independent of age, gender or body mass index (BMI). Murphy and colleagues[14] demonstrated that age did not produce a significant clinical difference in SF-12 score in patients undergoing TKA. Xu and colleagues"[15] 10-year follow-up study showed that overall, even patients with high BMI had satisfactory outcomes following TKAs and demonstrated an improvement in their preoperative pain and function scores.

The authors prospectively recruited patients for this study. It would have been interesting to analyze a matched group of patients undergoing a TKA without multimodal therapy. The SF-12 MCS, used in the authors' study, has been shown to be a useful screening tool to identify recent affective disorder.[16] The SF-12 is widely used, as it measures an individual's perception of physical and psychosocial aspects across 8 domains.[17] However, specific scoring systems looking at motivation, anxiety, and depression would also have helped in further understanding the role these factors play in influencing outcome after TKA. Long-term studies will be useful in understanding the role of these factors.

The multimodal intervention classes were available to all patients. The emphasis was on periarticular muscle strengthening, core muscle strengthening, education, and dietitian help. Information, guidance, and encouragement to adhere to self-management in the community were the focus.

A relationship between pain and outcomes was difficult to draw. Age, sex, or BMI did not seem to influence the outcome in these patients. This is consistent with other studies, although the influence of BMI is contested.[18–20] The importance of mental health in predicting pain and functional outcomes of joint replacement surgery has also been shown in these studies.

Psychological distress measured by the mental health score of the 36-Item Short Form Survey (SF-36) has been shown by 1 group to predict greater WOMAC pain and joint dysfunction scores following knee arthroplasty.[11] Studies have also highlighted the role of psychosocial health, motivation, and perception of illness on outcome after TKA.[21,22]

Depressive symptoms and anxiety were associated with pain and reduced function 5 years after TKAs.[6] The only meta-analysis published to date clearly showed a link between existing preoperative psychological disorders and the likelihood of a less-than-desired outcome after TKA.[23]

Scott and colleagues[3] found that the mental and physical component scores of the 12-Item Short Form Survey (SF-12) and pain to be independent predictors of satisfaction. Having positive expectations that one is going to have a good outcome, decreased pain, and improved function were found to be consistently related to improved satisfaction postoperatively.[18] Another study of revision TKA patients highlighted the influence of the perception of helplessness on outcomes after surgery.[24] Furthermore, a recent randomized control study focusing on patient expectations showed that these might be managed through patient education. The authors compared standard education versus e-learning and found that the e-learning group had better KSS (Knee Society Score) symptom scores. Surprisingly, despite these improved scores, it did not lessen the risk of not meeting their expected outcome.[25]

This study adds to this existing knowledge and also demonstrates that intervening by means of a nonoperative multimodal program positively impacts the symptoms of osteoarthritis and psychosocial health.

The authors are aware there may be other factors that confound their results, including technical challenges during the procedure itself. Although this was not taken into account in their study, the authors did not have any intra- or immediate postoperative complications.

SUMMARY

Osteoarthritis of the knee is a significant health problem associated with a long-term physical disability. Although the results of TKA for osteoarthritis of the knee are encouraging, there seems to be a cohort of patients not satisfied with the outcome. Several preoperative factors influence this finding. However, although the indication for TKA remains a clinical decision, the authors believe that preintervention with multimodal education and physiotherapy helps optimize the results of TKA in some patients. The authors have shown that multimodal therapy does improve PROMs in both patients diagnosed with osteoarthritis and those who proceed to a TKA. This contributes to data published to try and improve outcomes in patients undergoing a TKA. Perhaps it also gives patients an insight into the likelihood of outcomes and the timing of surgery. With time, conducting more focused, well-designed studies, augmented with data from the psychosocial analysis may enable surgeons to stratify and identify patients who are more likely to have a satisfactory outcome following TKA.

CLINICAL CARE POINTS

Multimodal therapy classes on the mental subscale of SF12 are relevant to outcome after primary TKA. Evidence demonstrates multimodal therapy in patients undergoing TKA positively impacts the outcome.

The number of TKAs will continue to rise, and patient education aimed at optimizing patients physically and psychosocially will be essential. Therefore there is scope for developing a specific robust scoring system, particularly for evaluating psychosocial domains that have not previously addressed well.

DISCLOSURE

The authors have nothing to disclose.

REFERENCES

1. Brittain R, Young E, Mccormack V, et al. 16th annual report 2019: National Joint Registry for England, Wales, Northern Ireland and the Isle of Man. 2019. Available at: https://www.hqip.org.uk/wp-content/uploads/2018/11/NJR-15th-Annual-Report-2018.pdf. Accessed January 3, 2020.
2. Evans JT, Evans JP, Walker RW, et al. How long does a hip replacement last? A systematic review and meta-analysis of case series and national registry reports with more than 15 years of follow-up. Lancet 2019.
3. Scott CEH, Howie CR, MacDonald D, et al. Predicting dissatisfaction following total knee replacement. J Bone Joint Surg Br 2010.
4. Brander VA, Stulberg SD, Adams AD, et al. Ranawat award paper: predicting total knee replacement pain. Clin Orthop Relat Res 2003.
5. Wylde V, Dieppe P, Hewlett S, et al. Total knee replacement: Is it really an effective procedure for all? Knee 2007;14(6):417–23.
6. Brander V, Gondek S, Martin E, et al. The John Insall award: pain and depression influence outcome 5 years after knee replacement surgery. Clin Orthop Relat Res 2007. https://doi.org/10.1097/BLO.0b013e318126c032.
7. Ayers DC, Franklin PD, Ploutz-Snyder R, et al. Total knee replacement outcome and coexisting physical and emotional illness. Clin Orthop Relat Res 2005.
8. Lingard EA, Katz JN, Wright EA, et al. Predicting the outcome of total knee arthroplasty. J Bone Joint Surg Am 2004;86(10):2179–86.
9. Faller H, Kirschner S, König A. Psychological distress predicts functional outcomes at three and twelve months after total knee arthroplasty. Gen Hosp Psychiatry 2003. https://doi.org/10.1016/S0163-8343(03)00062-8.
10. Fortin PR, Clarke AE, Joseph L, et al. Outcomes of total hip and knee replacement: Preoperative functional status predicts outcomes at six months after surgery. Arthritis Rheum 1999;42(8):1722–8.
11. Lingard EA, Riddle DL. Impact of psychological distress on pain and function following knee arthroplasty. J Bone Joint Surg Am 2007.
12. Hanusch BC, O'Connor DB, Ions P, et al. Effects of psychological distress and perceptions of illness on recovery from total knee replacement. Bone Joint J 2014. https://doi.org/10.1302/0301-620X.96B2.31136.
13. Patel S, Hossain FS, Paton B, et al. The effects of a non-operative multimodal programme on osteoarthritis of the knee. Ann R Coll Surg Engl 2010.
14. Murphy BPD, Dowsey MM, Spelman T, et al. The impact of older age on patient outcomes following primary total knee arthroplasty. Bone Joint J 2018.
15. Xu S, Chen JY, Lo NN, et al. The influence of obesity on functional outcome and quality of life after total knee arthroplasty. Bone Joint J 2018; 100B(5):579–83.
16. Vilagut G, Forero CG, Pinto-Meza A, et al. The mental component of the short-form 12 health survey (SF-12) as a measure of depressive disorders in the general population: Results with three alternative scoring methods. Value Health 2013.
17. Hampton SN, Wells JE, Nakonezny PA, et al. Pain catastrophising, anxiety, and depression in hip pathology. Bone Joint J 2019;101 B(7):800–7.
18. Anderson JG, Wixson RL, Tsai D, et al. Functional outcome and patient satisfaction in total knee patients over the age of 75. J Arthroplasty 1996.
19. Noble PC, Conditt MA, Cook KF, et al. The John Insall Award: patient expectations affect satisfaction with total knee arthroplasty. Clin Orthop Relat Res 2006.
20. Gandhi R, Davey JR, Mahomed NN. Predicting patient dissatisfaction following joint replacement surgery. J Rheumatol 2008. https://doi.org/10.3899/jrheum.080295.
21. Botha-Scheepers S, Riyazi N, Kroon HM, et al. Activity limitations in the lower extremities in patients with osteoarthritis: the modifying effects of illness perceptions and mental health. Osteoarthr Cartil 2006.
22. Kaptein AA, Bijsterbosch J, Scharloo M, et al. Using the common sense model of illness perceptions to examine osteoarthritis change: a 6-year longitudinal study. Health Psychol 2010.
23. Sorel JC, Veltman ES, Honig A, et al. The influence of preoperative psychological distress on pain and function after total knee arthroplasty: a systematic review and meta-analysis. Bone Joint J 2019; 101B(1):7–14.

24. Venkataramanan V, Gignac MA, Dunbar M, et al. The importance of perceived helplessness and emotional health in understanding the relationship among pain, function, and satisfaction following revision knee replacement surgery. Osteoarthr Cartil 2013.

25. MacDonald SJ, Culliton SE, Bryant D, et al. A randomized controlled trial to establish realistic patient expectations following total knee replacement surgery. Bone Joint J 2018;4268.https://online.boneandjoint.org.uk/doi/abs/10.1302/1358-992X.2018.12.064.

Trauma

Ski and Snowboard - Related Orthopedic Injuries

Zachary L. Telgheder, MD*, Brian J. Kistler, MD

KEYWORDS

• Ski • Snowboard • Trauma • Sports • Knee

KEY POINTS

- Skiing and snowboarding are popular winter sports, and participation continues to increase.
- Injuries to the entire musculoskeletal system are described with both sports, with lower extremity injuries more common in skiing and upper extremity injuries more common in snowboarding.
- Spinal injuries are described in both skiing and snowboarding, with injuries reported about the cervical, thoracic, and lumbar spine.
- Both sports demonstrate unique injuries related to their environment, pathomechanics, and equipment, such as hip dislocations, anterior cruciate ligament injuries, fractures of the lateral process of the talus, and thumb ulnar collateral ligament injuries.
- Recognition of risk factors and injury patterns can help aid in diagnosis and treatment of these potentially complex orthopedic injuries.

INTRODUCTION

Skiing and snowboarding are popular winter sports that attract children and adults alike. In 2018 to 2019, an estimated 10.3 million people participated in skiing and snowboarding in the United States.[1] This represents the highest estimated total number of participants since the National Ski Areas Association began tracking data in the 1996 to 1997 season. The overall number of skier and snowboarder visits during the 2018 to 2019 season exceeded 59 million, representing an 11% increase over the 2017 to 2018 winter season.[2] Prior reports have indicated that the rates of injury sustained during snowboarding are up to 3 times higher than those sustained while skiing.[3,4] As awareness of injury patterns and preventive measures, particularly the use of helmets, has improved, the overall rate of ski and snowboard-related injuries has decreased.[5] Despite this, there are numerous well-described musculoskeletal injuries related

to the speed, movement patterns, and unique equipment utilized in these activities.[6,7] Furthermore, the pattern of injury associated with these sports has evolved over time.[3] A thorough understanding of the injuries sustained during skiing and snowboarding is essential to the orthopedic surgeon, as all anatomic areas and systems are potentially at risk with participation in these sports (Table 1).

Epidemiology

The earliest comprehensive report of injuries sustained while skiing was documented in Sun Valley, Idaho, with a reported ski injury incidence rate of 7.6 injuries per 1000 skier-days from 1952 to 1957.[8–10] Other studies examining injury rates dating back to the 1960s similarly demonstrated high rates of injury.[11] More recent studies examining rates of injury have demonstrated lower incidence of injury than first reported. Davidson and Laliotis reviewed 24,340 injuries in Alpine skiers from 1983 to 1992 in California, and found

---

Funded by: SUNY.

Department of Orthopedic Surgery, SUNY Upstate Medical University, 750 East Adams Street, Suite 4400, Syracuse, NY 13210, USA

* Corresponding author.

E-mail address: ztelgheder@gmail.com

Table 1
Common injuries sustained by skiers and snowboarders

Common Ski and Snowboard - Related Orthopedic Injuries		
Common Skiing Injuries	Common Snowboarding Injuries	Notable Injuries Sustained in Both Sports
Knee ligamentous injuries (ACL, MCL)	Wrist injuries (distal radius fractures)	Spinal Fractures
Hand and thumb injuries (thumb UCL injuries)	Shoulder injuries (clavicle fractures, glenohumeral dislocations)	Sacral fractures, pubic rami fractures
Tibial shaft fractures	Foot and ankle injuries (ankle fractures, talus fractures)	Hip dislocations and fracture-dislocations

the overall injury rate to be 2.6 injuries per 1000 skier days.[12] This rate of injury is comparable to other large-scale studies, demonstrating rates of injury from 1.43 to 2.8 injuries per 1000 skier days.[5,13,14] According to the National Ski Areas Association 10-year interval injury study released in 2010, the weighted skiing incident rate was 2.5 injuries per 1000 visits, and the weighted snowboard incident rate was 6.1 injuries per 1000 visits, with both sports demonstrating lower injury rates than in 2000.[5]

In evaluation of distribution of injuries by gender, rates of injury have varied among prior studies. Davidson and Laliotis noted an equal distribution of injuries among male and female patients in their series.[12] In a review of 17,914 skiing injuries, Burtscher and colleagues[13] noted that 52% of all injuries sustained were by female patients. Several other reports have noted a higher cumulative incidence of injuries in male patients, particularly regarding snowboarding injuries.[3,15–18]

It is important to note that children and adolescents represent a substantial portion of skiers and snowboarders, and prior epidemiologic studies have demonstrated that young age is a significant predictor of injury during participation.[19] The overall incidence of injury in children during skiing and snowboarding requiring emergency department visitation is estimated to be 15 to 20 injuries per 1000 visits.[20] As with studies evaluating injuries in adults, children and adolescents injured while snowboarding are more likely to be boys.[21]

Injury Patterns
Although both skiing and snowboarding pose risk of injury, there are key differences in the anatomic distribution of injuries sustained. Both skiers and snowboarders are at risk for lower extremity injury; however, the overall incidence of lower extremity injury is higher in skiing than in snowboarding.[3,12,22–24] In contrast, the rate of

upper extremity injury is higher in snowboarders than in skiers.[3,12,22] Snowboarding participants are at higher risk of wrist, shoulder, and clavicle injuries than skiers.[3,22,23,25]

With regards to injuries of the spinal column, overall injury rates appear to be higher among skiers when compared with snowboarders.[26–28] Prior studies demonstrate that the lumbar spine is more commonly injured during snowboarding when compared with spinal injuries sustained while skiing. De Roulet and colleagues[7] noted that thoracic spine injuries were most common among skiers, while Hubbard and colleagues[29] found that the cervical spine was the most injured spinal segment; both demonstrated that the lumbar spine was most injured in snowboarders.

Although the focus of this article is orthopedic injuries related to skiing and snowboarding, it is important to note that multiple-system injuries are common in these sports. In their review of Alpine skiing injuries, Davey and colleagues[30] reported a 13% overall incidence of head and neck injuries, and a 5% incidence of thoracoabdominal injuries. Sacco and colleagues[22] noted a 17% incidence of head and neck injuries and an 18% incidence of thoracic and abdominal injuries in their study of ski and snowboard-related injuries. Furthermore, Levy and Smith noted that head injuries comprised 28% and 33.5% of injuries in skiers and snowboarders, respectively.[26] Although the definitive treatment of these injuries may be outside the scope of the orthopedic surgeon, it is imperative that the orthopedic surgeon be aware of the considerations of the polytraumatized patient and understand the implications of these multiple-system injuries on the overall care of the patient.

SPECIFIC INJURIES
Spinal Injuries
The reported overall incidence of injuries to the spinal column in skiers and snowboarders ranges

from 1.4% to 20.7%, with reported incidence of injury in patients sustaining severe injuries as high as 28.9%.[23,29,31] The repetitive jumping and landing seen in snowboarding and freestyle skiing have contributed to higher rates of spinal injury in these patient populations.[31,32] As mentioned previously, higher rates of lumbar spine injuries have been noted in snowboarders, although location of spinal injuries has varied among skiers.[7,29]

Among spinal fractures, vertebral body fractures are the most common injuries, with various fracture patterns reported. In a series examining spinal injuries in skiers and snowboarders, Tarazi and colleagues[32] noted that burst fractures were the most common spinal fractures in skiers and snowboarders, comprising 60% and 63.2%, respectively, of fractures reported. An example of a lumbar burst fracture sustained during snowboarding is seen in **Fig. 1**. Compression fractures represented 40% of spinal fractures in skiers, and 36.8% of spinal fractures in snowboarders. Cervical facet fractures represented 11.1% of fractures in skiers, compared with only 3.7% in snowboarders.[32] In contrast, Yamakawa and colleagues[31] found that among 91 skiers with spinal fractures, 85.7% were compression fractures, and 14.3% were burst fractures, and noted that 91% of fractures in 252 snowboarders were compression fractures. Both series demonstrated that sacrococcygeal, spinous process fractures, odontoid fractures, and cervical tear drop fractures were relatively rare.[31,32] In their series of 61 skiing-related and 51 snowboard-related thoracolumbar fractures,

Gertzbein and colleagues[33] found that compression fractures were the most common fracture types in both sports, comprising 63.9% of fractures in skiers and 80.4% of fractures in snowboarders. It was also found that distraction and rotational-type fractures were relatively rare, with 8.2% and 1.6% of ski-related fractures demonstrating these subtypes.

The rates of spinal cord and neurologic injury among skiers and snowboarders also vary in the reported literature. Spinal cord injury is most associated with injuries of the cervical spine, with rates as high as 24% reported.[31–34] In a retrospective series of 19 patients with surgically treated traumatic spinal injuries, Masuda and colleagues[35] reported that the predominant site of neurologic injury was the thoracolumbar junction, with 13 of 19 patients in their series sustaining injury at this level. The authors found that fracture-dislocations were the most common vertebral injury type, and in their series 63.2% of patients presented with either Frankel grade A or B paralysis.[35] Although neurologic injuries are most often associated with fractures, other mechanisms of injury, including traumatic cervical disc rupture, have also been reported.[36] Given the incidence of spinal column injury in skiers and snowboarders, it is important that surgeons have a high index of suspicion for neurologic injuries in these athletes.

Injuries of the Pelvis, Acetabulum, and Hip
The overall rate of pelvic and acetabular trauma related to skiing and snowboarding is low in the reported literature. Hasler and colleagues noted

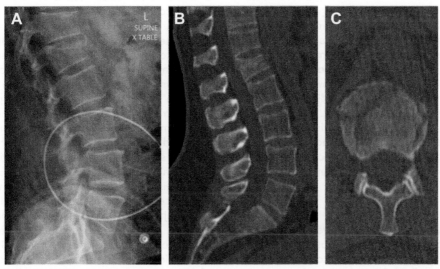

Fig. 1. Images of a lumbar burst fracture sustained by a snowboarder landing from a jump. (*A*) Demonstrates a lateral radiograph showing a burst fracture of the L1 vertebral body. (*B*, *C*) Demonstrate computed tomography scans obtained at the time of injury.

that pelvic injuries represented 8% of all injuries in their series of patients sustaining major injuries while skiing or snowboarding, after excluding patients with isolated injuries of the extremities.[37] Aitken and colleagues noted only 2 lateral compression-type pelvic ring injuries, representing 1.9% of ski and snowboard-related fractures.[38] In a series of 145 patients with pelvic fractures sustained during snowboarding, Ogawa and colleagues[39] found that these fractures represented 2.0% of all fractures sustained while snowboarding. In this series, 85.5% of pelvic ring injuries were classified as type A per the Tile Classification, representing stable injuries; those who sustained Tile type B or C injuries were more likely to sustain their pelvic ring injury after a jump or a collision, while those with a stable injury were more likely to be injured during a fall. In addition, the rate of associated injuries was 33.3% in the unstable injury group, compared with 18.5% in the stable injury group, highlighting the more severe nature of these injuries.[39] The authors reported that 46.9% of fractures were isolated fractures of the pubic bone or the ischium; 24.1% were isolated sacral fractures, 15.9% combined injuries involving multiple segments of the pelvic ring, and 10.3% were acetabular fractures. The authors note that consideration should be given to sacral fractures as a cause of buttock pain in snowboarders given their 24.1% incidence in this study and their relative overall rarity.[39]

Traumatic hip dislocations have also been reported because of skiing and snowboarding. A retrospective report of 86 patients with traumatic hip dislocations treated in Davos demonstrated that 66% of injuries were sustained during Alpine skiing, with 22% of those sustaining traumatic hip dislocations demonstrating associated injuries.[40] Matsumoto and colleagues[41] found that hip dislocations were 5 times more common in snowboarders than skiers, and that anterior hip dislocations were significantly more frequent during snowboarding. Although rare, this injury represents a surgical emergency requiring prompt diagnosis and reduction, and orthopedic surgeons should be aware that this injury has been reported during these activities.

Lower Extremity Injuries

When evaluating specific lower extremity injuries, sprains and ligamentous injuries about the knee are the most common injuries noted.[3,12,15,21–23] Prior epidemiologic studies have demonstrated that knee injuries represent from 27% to 40.8% of injuries sustained by skiers.[12,13,15,16,42,43] In comparison with 1.7% of snowboarding injuries, Kim and colleagues[3] noted that injuries to the anterior cruciate ligament comprised 17.2% of all skiing injuries. There are multiple described mechanisms of anterior cruciate ligament (ACL) injuries in skiers. A valgus external rotational force secondary to a fall forward over the fixed inner edge of the front ski has been described, as well as the phantom foot phenomenon, in which the skier falls backwards as the downhill knee is subjected to an internal rotation force while flexed.[15,44,45] A third proposed mechanism includes an anterior-directed force upon the tibia during landing with the knee in extension because of the position of the ski boot relative to the tibia.[46] In a review of video footage of 20 ACL injuries sustained during World Cup Alpine skiing, Bere and colleagues found that 50% of injuries were related to a slip-catch mechanism, in which a skier sustained a valgus and internal rotation force about the knee after the inner edge of the outer ski became caught in the snow during extension to regain balance.[47] The authors also noted that the ski bindings failed to release in 17 of 20 subjects in their study.[47] Although less common in snowboarders, a proposed mechanism of ACL injury involves eccentric quadriceps contraction upon the flexed knee after landing on a flat surface, resulting in forced internal rotation of the knee.[48] All the aforementioned proposed mechanisms are unique to skiing and snowboarding, because of the distinctive equipment and movement patterns found in the sport.

As is expected with valgus and rotational-directed forces about the knee, concomitant medial collateral ligament (MCL) and meniscal injuries are common in skiers (Fig. 2). In a review of 28 elite Alpine ski racing athletes undergoing ACL reconstruction, Jordan and colleagues[49] found that 82% of knees demonstrated concomitant injury during surgical treatment. In this series, the authors found that 61% of patients demonstrated concomitant meniscal injuries; 54% demonstrated chondral lesions, and 32% sustained multiligamentous injuries, with 7 of 9 patients sustaining ipsilateral MCL injuries. The authors also found that 22% of subjects underwent revision ACL reconstruction after their index procedure, underscoring the complexity of these injuries.[49] These results are consistent with the findings of Duncan and colleagues,[50] who retrospectively found that 159 of 315 skiers undergoing ACL reconstruction sustained a total of 170 meniscal tears, with 83% of the tears located in the lateral meniscus.

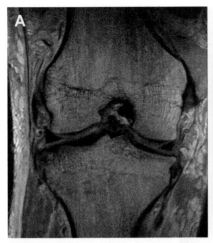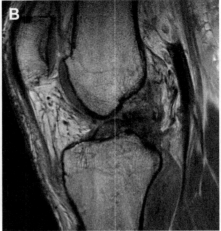

Fig. 2. MRI of combined ACL, MCL and meniscal injuries sustained by a 32-year-old skier after a fall. *A* and *B* demonstrate complete ruptures of the anterior cruciate ligament and a grade III Injury of the medial collateral ligament. The patient ultimately underwent staged ligamentous reconstruction.

Fractures about the tibia are also common in this patient population. In a review of 372 fractures of the tibia sustained while skiing or snowboarding, Stenroos and colleagues[51] found that fractures of the tibial shaft were the most common fracture in skiers, and that proximal tibia fractures were most common in snowboarders. Snowboarders were more likely to sustain AO type C fractures of the tibia than skiers in their study, and the overall prevalence of proximal tibia fractures was higher in adults than children.[51] Pätzold and colleagues[52] noted an increased prevalence of proximal tibia fractures between 2007 and 2010, and found that AO type C proximal tibia fractures in skiers were associated with higher age, greater body mass index (BMI), higher skiing speed, icy conditions, and skill level compared with type A and B fractures.

Although the overall incidence of lower extremity injuries is higher in skiers, injuries of the foot and ankle are more common in snowboarders, with foot and ankle injuries representing 17.1% of all injuries in snowboarders in 1 study.[53] Most ankle injuries were sprains (52%) and ankle fractures (44%), while 57% of foot injuries were fractures.[53] Patton and colleagues[54] demonstrated that compared with skiers, snowboarders were more likely to sustain ankle fractures; they noted that most of these fractures were about the left, or lead foot in snowboarders. Fractures of the tibial plafond have been described during skiing, secondary to vertical impact and axial load through the plafond as the skier lands during jumping.[55]

An injury unique to snowboarding is a fracture of the lateral talar process, colloquially referred to as the snowboarder's fracture. Kirkparick and colleagues[53] found that these fractures represented 34% of all fractures about the ankle in their prospective study of 3213 snowboarding injuries. The mechanism of injury was initially proposed to be forced hindfoot inversion with axial loading during ankle dorsiflexion; however, cadaveric studies and more recent clinical retrospective studies have shown that hindfoot eversion in concert with dorsiflexion and axial load is more likely to produce this distinct fracture.[56,57]

Valderrabano and colleagues[57] evaluated 20 patients sustaining fractures of the lateral process of the talus at a mean of 42 months after injury. The authors found that in patients with type II injuries with greater than 2 mm of displacement, American Orthopedic Foot and Ankle Society Ankle-Hindfoot Scale scores were higher in those undergoing operative treatment compared with nonoperative treatment (**Fig. 3**).[57] The authors also noted that all 4 of the patients who did not return to the same level of activity prior to injury underwent nonoperative treatment, forming the basis for their conclusion that primary surgical treatment led to improved outcomes in displaced, type II fractures.[57]

Upper Extremity Injuries

Injuries about the shoulder girdle are well-described in skiers and in snowboarders, and occur more frequently among snowboarders. Kocher and Feagin found that injuries to the shoulder girdle comprised 39.1% of upper extremity injuries and 11.4% of all injuries in a series of 3451 Alpine skiing injuries.[58] The authors found that 93.9% of shoulder injuries

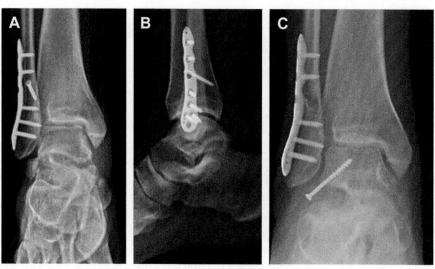

Fig. 3. (*A, B*) Demonstrate PA and lateral radiographs of the right ankle in a snowboarder who sustained a displaced type II lateral process of the talus fracture after a fall. The patient had previously sustained an unstable lateral malleolus fracture while snowboarding treated with open reduction and internal fixation. (*C*) PA radiograph demonstrating union after open reduction and internal fixation.

were related to falls, and found that the most common shoulder girdle injuries were rotator cuff strains (24.2%), acromioclavicular joint separations (19.6%), and clavicle fractures (10.9%).[58] Kim and colleagues[3] found that injuries about the shoulder represented 11.7% of all reported injuries in snowboarders, with clavicle fractures representing 4% of snowboarding injuries. With regards to clavicle fractures, Kim and colleagues[3] found that a higher proportion of clavicle fractures were sustained in terrain parks, with 33.7% of clavicle fractures sustained during jumping. In a review of 2742 snowboarders and 361 skiers with upper extremity injuries, Matsumoto and colleagues[59] found that glenohumeral dislocations represented 5.5% and 6.5% of upper extremity injuries in skiers and snowboarders, respectively. It was also noted that clavicle fractures were the most common upper extremity fracture sustained while skiing, and that elbow dislocations were rare but significantly more common in snowboarders, representing 30% of dislocations as opposed to just 3% in skiers.[59]

Injuries about the wrist are also common injuries and are more frequently observed in snowboarders. Sasaki and colleagues[60] reported that wrist injuries represented 36.4% of upper extremity injuries in snowboarders, compared with 9.1% of upper extremity injuries in skiers. They also found that physeal fractures of the distal radius were 2 times more prevalent among snowboarders, and that AO type A3, B, and C

fractures were more than twice as prevalent in snowboarders, signifying greater fracture complexity.[60] In a study of 7430 snowboard-related injuries, Idzikowski and colleagues[25] noted that injuries to the wrist comprised 21.6% of all injuries, representing the most common injury pattern in their series. Although most of these wrist injuries were distal radius fractures, the authors did note that perilunate dislocations and lunate fracture-dislocations represented 2% of wrist injuries in their series, again demonstrating the substantial energy that can be imparted on the wrist during snowboarding.[25]

Injuries about the hand are also encountered in both skiing and snowboarding, with different injury patterns noted between the 2 sports. Idzikowski and colleagues[25] noted that injuries to the hand represented 8.4% of upper extremity injuries in snowboarders, with 50% of hand injuries representing fractures. The authors also found that injuries to the ulnar collateral ligament (UCL) of the thumb metacarpophalangeal joint represented only 1.8% of hand injuries in their series.[25] This is notable, because thumb UCL injuries represent a common injury among skiers, with this injury often referred to as a skier's thumb. Van Dommelen and Zvirbulis noted that thumb UCL injuries account for nearly 80% of upper extremity injuries sustained by skiers.[61] The mechanism of injury involves forced thumb metacarpophalangeal joint abduction and extension as the skier's hand is directed forward while grabbing a ski pole, either with the pole fixed in the snow or during a fall.[62] Although this injury is common among skiers, this injury may be under-reported because of lack of perceived severity by skiers.[63] Because of this, a thorough history evaluating for injury mechanism and physical examination are critical for the treating surgeon. In cases of suspected thumb UCL injury, ultrasound represents a cost-effective and efficacious diagnostic test, with 92% sensitivity and 99% positive predictive value reported.[64]

SUMMARY

Although both skiing and snowboarding are popular winter sports, they both demonstrate substantial injury risk. Even though both sports demonstrate different patterns of injury, available evidence shows that the axial skeleton and extremities are at risk for injury. Knowledge of the injury patterns inherent to skiing and snowboarding allows the treating orthopedic surgeon to diagnose and treat these potentially complex injuries accurately and efficiently. Future research regarding skiing and snowboarding-related injuries will likely emphasize optimization of equipment and injury prevention to reduce the incidence of traumatic injury related to these sports.

CLINICS CARE POINTS

According to multiple sources, including the National Ski Areas Association 10-year interval injury study released in 2010, the incidence of injury during skiing and snowboarding is approximately 2.5 injuries per 1000 skier days.[5,11–14] Although orthopedic injuries to the upper and lower extremities are common with these sports, the incidence of lower extremity injuries is higher in skiing, and the incidence of upper extremity injuries is higher in snowboarding.[3,12,22]

Vertebral body fractures represent the most common spinal injury in skiers and snowboarders, with injuries to the lumbar spine more common among snowboarders.[7,23,29] Injuries of the ACL are the most common orthopedic injury found in skiers, with ACL injuries comprising up to 17% of all injuries among these athletes.[3]

Displaced type II fractures of the lateral process of the talus, an injury encountered in snowboarders, demonstrate improved outcomes with operative treatment compared with nonoperative treatment.[57] Thumb ulnar collateral ligament injuries are common in skiers, and are often sustained forced thumb metacarpophalangeal joint abduction and extension as the skier's hand is directed forward while grabbing a ski pole, either with the pole fixed in the snow or during a fall.[62]

DISCLOSURE

The authors have nothing to disclose.

REFERENCES

1. National Ski Areas Association. Estimated snowsports participants, snowsports visits, and average visits per participant U.S. Visitors to U.S. Resorts, 1996/97 – 2018/19. Lakewood (CO): National Ski Areas Association; 2019.
2. National Ski Areas Association. Estimated U.S. snowsports visits by region, 1978/79 – 2018/19. Lakewood (CO): National Ski Areas Association; 2019.
3. Kim S, Endres NK, Johnson RJ, et al. Snowboarding injuries: trends over time and comparisons with alpine skiing injuries. Am J Sports Med 2012;40(4):770–6.
4. Made C, Elmqvist LG. A 10-year study of snowboard injuries in Lapland Sweden. Scand J Med Sci Sports 2004;14(2):128–33.
5. Shealy JE, Ettlinger CF, Johnson RJ. 2010/2011 NSAA 10-year interval injury study. J ASTM Int 2013;(STP1582):93–111.
6. Diebert MC, Aronsson DD, Johnson RJ, et al. Skiing injuries in children, adolescents, and adults. J Bone Joint Surg Am 1998;80:25–32.
7. de Roulet A, Inaba K, Strumwasser A, et al. Severe injuries associated with skiing and snowboarding: a national trauma data bank study. J Trauma Acute Care Surg 2017;82:781–6.
8. Earle AS, Moritz JR, Saviers GB. Ski injuries. JAMA 1962;180:285–8.
9. Moritz JR. Ski injuries. Am J Surg 1959;98:493–505.
10. Tapper EM. Ski injuries from 1939 to 1976: The Sun Valley experience. Am J Sports Med 1978;6:114–21.
11. Sherry E, Fenelon L. Trends in skiing injury type and rates in Australia-A review of 22,261 injuries over 27 years in the Snowy Mountains. Med J Aust 1991;155:513–5.
12. Davidson TM, Laliotis AT. Alpine skiing injuries—a nine-year study. West J Med 1996;164:310–4.
13. Burtscher M, Gatterer H, Flatz M, et al. Effects of modern ski equipment on the overall injury rate and the pattern of injury location in Alpine skiing. Clin J Sport Med 2008;18:355–7.
14. Bianchi G, Brügger O, Niemann S. Skiing and snowboarding in Switzerland: trends in injury and fatality rates over time. In: Scher I, Greenwald R, Petrone

N, editors. Snow sports trauma and safety. Cham, Switzerland: Springer Open; 2017. pp. 29–39.

15. Sulheim S, Holme I, Rodven A, et al. Risk factors for injuries in Alpine skiing, telemark skiing and snowboarding—case-control study. Br J Sports Med 2011;45:1303–9.

16. Ruedl G, Kopp M, Sommersacher R, et al. Factors associated with injuries occurred on slope intersections and in snow parks compared to on-slope injuries. Accid Anal Prev 2013;50:1221–5.

17. Stenroos A, Handolin L. Incidence of recreational alpine skiing and snowboarding injuries: six years' experience in the largest ski resort in Finland. Scand J Surg 2015;104:127–31.

18. Pino EC, Colville MR. Snowboard injuries. Am J Sports Med 1989;17:778–81.

19. Cadman R, Macnab A. Age and gender: two epidemiological factors in skiing and snowboarding injury. ski. Trauma Saf Tenth Vol. 100 Barr Harbor Drive, PO Box C700, West Conshohocken (PA) 19428–2959: Injury Prevention 1996 [58–58–8].

20. Xiang H, Kelleher K, Shields BJ, et al. Skiing- and snowboarding-related injuries treated in U.S. emergency departments, 2002. J Trauma 2005;58:112–8.

21. Polites S, Mao S, Glasgow A, et al. Safety on the slopes: ski versus snowboard injuries in children treated at United States trauma centers. J Pediatr Surg 2018;53:1024–7.

22. Sacco DE, Sartorelli DH, Vane DW. Evaluation of Alpine skiing and snowboarding injury in a northeastern state. J Trauma 1998;44:654–9.

23. Wasden CC, McIntosh SE, Keith DS, et al. An analysis of skiing and snowboarding injuries on Utah slopes. J Trauma 2009;67(5):1022–6.

24. Basques BA, Gardner EC, Samuel AM, et al. Injury patterns and risk factors for orthopaedic trauma from snowboarding and skiing: a national perspective. Knee Surg Sports Traumatol Arthrosc 2016; 26(7):1916–26.

25. Idzikowski JR, Janes PC, Abbott PJ. Upper extremity snowboarding injuries: ten-year results from the Colorado snowboard injury survey. Am J Sports Med 2000;28(6):825–32.

26. Levy AS, Smith RH. Neurologic injuries in skiers and snowboarders. Semin Neurol 2000;20:233–45.

27. Franz T, Hasler RM, Benneker L, et al. Severe spinal injuries in alpine skiing and snowboarding: a 6-year review of a tertiary trauma Centre for the Bernese Alps ski resorts, Switzerland. Br J Sports Med 2008;42(1):55–8.

28. Prall JA, Winston KR, Brennan R. Severe snowboarding injuries. Injury 1995;26:539–42.

29. Hubbard ME, Jewell RP, Dumont TM, et al. Spinal injury patterns among skiers and snowboarders. Neurosurg Focus 2011;31(5):E8.

30. Davey A, Endres NK, Johnson RJ, et al. Alpine skiing injuries. Sports Health 2019;11(1):18–26.

31. Yamakawa H, Murase S, Sakai H, et al. Spinal injuries in snowboarders: risk of jumping as an integral part of snowboarding. J Trauma 2001;50(6):1101–5.

32. Tarazi F, Dvorak MF, Wing PC. Spinal injuries in skiers and snowboarders. Am J Sports Med 1999; 27(2):177–80.

33. Gertzbein SD, Khoury D, Bullington A, et al. Thoracic and lumbar fractures associated with skiing and snowboarding injuries according to the AO comprehensive classification. Am J Sports Med 2012;40(8):1750–4.

34. Bigdon SF, Geweiss J, Hoppe S, et al. Spinal Injury in alpine winter sports: a review. Scand J Trauma Resusc Emerg Med 2019;27:69.

35. Masuda T, Miyamoto K, Wakahara K, et al. Clinical outcomes of surgical treatments for traumatic spinal injuries due to snowboarding. Asian Spine J 2015;9(1):90–8.

36. Ecker TM, Kleinschmidt M, Martinolli L, et al. Clinical presentation of a traumatic cervical spine disc rupture in alpine sports: a case report. Scand J Trauma Resusc Emerg Med 2008;16:14.

37. Hasler RM, Schmucker U, Evangelopoulos DS, et al. Improving prehospital trauma management for skiers and snowboarders - need for on-slope triage? J Trauma Manag Outcomes 2011;5(1):5.

38. Aitken SA, Watson BS, Wood AM, et al. Sports-related fractures in South East Scotland: an analysis of 990 fractures. J Orthop Surg (Hong Kong) 2014;22:313–7.

39. Ogawa H, Sumi H, Sumi Y, et al. Pelvic fractures resulting from snowboarding. Am J Sports Med 2010;38(3):538–42.

40. Holzach P, Weymann A, Perren T, et al. Traumatic hip dislocations. Epidemiologic data at Davos Hospital and a multicenter study in Graubünden Canton. Z Unfallchir Versicherungsmed 1993;(Suppl 1):187–93.

41. Matsumoto K, Sumi H, Sumi Y, et al. An analysis of hip dislocations among snowboarders and skiers: a 10-year prospective study from 1992 to 2002. J Trauma 2003;55:946–8.

42. Patrick E, Cooper JG, Daniels J. Changes in skiing and snowboarding injury epidemiology and attitudes to safety in Big Sky, Montana, USA: a comparison of 2 cross-sectional studies in 1996 and 2013. Orthop J Sports Med 2015;3. 2325967115588280.

43. Johnson RJ, Ettlinger CF, Shealy JE. Skier injury trends—1972 to 2012. Paper presented at: Congress of the International Society of Skiing Safety; Bariloche, Patagonia, Argentina, August 5, 2013.

44. Hunter RE. Skiing injuries. Am J Sports Med 1999; 27:381–9.

45. Ettlinger CF, Johnson RJ, Shealy JE. A method to help reduce the risk of serious knee sprains incurred in alpine skiing. Am J Sports Med 1995; 23:531–7.

46. McConkey JP. Anterior cruciate ligament rupture in skiing. A new mechanism of injury. Am J Sports Med 1986;14:160–4.

47. Bere T, Flørenes TW, Krosshaug T, et al. Mechanisms of anterior cruciate ligament injury in World Cup alpine skiing: A systematic video analysis of 20 cases. Am J Sports Med 2011;39(7):1421–9.

48. Sachtleben TR. Snowboarding injuries. Curr Sports Med Rep 2011;10(6):340–4.

49. Jordan MJ, Doyle-Baker P, Heard M, et al. A retrospective analysis of concurrent pathology in ACL-reconstructed knees of elite alpine ski racers. Orthop J Sports Med 2017;5. 2325967117714756.

50. Duncan JB, Hunter R, Purnell M, et al. Meniscal injuries associated with acute anterior cruciate ligament tears in alpine skiers. Am J Sports Med 1995;23:170–2.

51. Stenroos A, Pakarinen H, Jalkanen J, et al. Tibial fractures in alpine skiing and snowboarding in Finland: a retrospective study on fracture types and injury mechanisms in 363 patients. Scand J Surg 2016;105:191–6.

52. Patzold R, Spiegl U, Wurster M, et al. Proximal tibial fractures sustained during alpine skiing—incidence and risk factors [in German]. Sportverletz Sportschaden 2013;27:207–11.

53. Kirkpatrick DP, Hunter RE, Janes PC, et al. The snowboarder's foot and ankle. Am J Sports Med 1998;26:271Y7.

54. Patton A, Bourne J, Theis JC. Patterns of lower limb fractures sustained during snowsports in Otago, New Zealand. N Z Med J 2010;123:20Y5.

55. Leach RE, Lower G. Ankle injuries in skiing. Clin Orthop Relat Res 1985;198:127–33.

56. Boon AJ, Smith J, Zobitz ME. Snowboarder's talus fracture Mechanism of injury. Am J Sports Med 2001;29(3):333–8.

57. Valderrabano V, Perren T, Ryf C, et al. Snowboarder's talus fracture: treatment outcome of 20 cases after 3.5 years. Am J Sports Med 2005;33: 871–80.

58. Kocher MS, Feagin JA Jr. Shoulder injuries during alpine skiing. Am J Sports Med 1996;24:665–9.

59. Matsumoto K, Miyamoto K, Sumi H, et al. Upper extremity injuries in snowboarding and skiing: a comparative study. Clin J Sport Med 2002;12:354–9.

60. Sasaki K, Takagi M, Kiyoshige Y, et al. Snowboarder's wrist: Its severity compared with Alpine skiing. J Trauma 1999;46(6):1059–61.

61. Van Dommelen BA, Zvirbulis RA. Upper extremity injuries in snow skiers. Am J Sports Med 1989; 17(6):751–3.

62. Keramidas E, Miller G. Adult hand injuries on artificial ski slopes. Ann Plast Surg 2005;55(4):357–8.

63. Hauser W. Experimental prospective skiing injury study. J ASTM Int 1989;(STP1022):18–24.

64. Chuter GS, Muwanga CL, Irwin LR. Ulnar collateral ligament injuries of the thumb: 10 years of surgical experience. Injury 2009;40(6):652–6.

Soft Tissue Injury Considerations in the Treatment of Tibial Plateau Fractures

John D. (JD) Adams Jr, MD[a],*,
Markus F. Loeffler, MD, MA[b]

KEYWORDS

- Tibial plateau • Soft tissue injury • Multiligamentous knee injury

---

KEY POINTS

- Tibial plateau fractures are complex bony and soft tissue injuries that require comprehensive evaluation and meticulous planning.
- Injuries to the soft tissue structures in tibial plateau fractures are often underestimated. Appropriate treatment of these associated injuries may be critical in obtaining good clinical outcomes; however, the literature is sparse.
- If possible, MRI should be used as the advanced imaging modality of choice in tibial plateau fractures, because it provides excellent bony detail while also providing important information regarding the soft tissue structures of the knee.

INTRODUCTION

Tibial plateau fracture is a broad term encompassing a variable presentation of injury. These intraarticular fractures range from simple split patterns to highly complex patterns with varying extension into the metaphysis or diaphysis of the tibia. This fracture accounts for approximately 1% of all fractures and affects adults of all ages. However, higher energy mechanisms are typically associated with younger age groups.[1,2] Historically, treatment plans for tibial plateau fractures have focused on restoring the bony architecture. We now understand that most of these injuries affect not only the bone but also the soft tissue. This article focuses on how the soft tissue should be considered in the treatment of these complex injuries.

NATURE OF THE PROBLEM

In recent years, there has been an increased interest in soft tissue injuries associated with tibial plateau fractures, likely driven by continued poor outcomes. Despite our best efforts at reconstruction of the proximal tibia, patients can continue to have pain, deformity, instability, wound complications, and decreased range of motion.[2–5]

Although ideal treatment of these complex injuries continues to evolve over time, the emphasis on the preservation and appropriate handling of the soft tissues has remained a principle of tibial plateau fracture management.[2,4,6,7] In the past, this emphasis has primarily focused on surgical timing and the inflammatory response of the soft tissue envelope

---

[a] Department of Orthopedic Surgery, Division of Orthopedic Trauma, Prisma Health, Greenville Memorial Medical Hospital, 701 Grove Road, 2nd Floor Support Tower, Greenville, SC 29605, USA; [b] Department of Orthopedic Surgery, Prisma Health, Greenville Memorial Medical Hospital, 701 Grove Road, 2nd Floor Support Tower, Greenville, SC 29605, USA
* Corresponding author.
E-mail addresses: Jd.Adams@prismahealth.org; johnweinlein@gmail.com

Orthop Clin N Am 51 (2020) 471–479
https://doi.org/10.1016/j.ocl.2020.06.003
0030-5898/20/© 2020 Elsevier Inc. All rights reserved.

before definitive management. More recently, there has been an increasing focus on specific soft tissue injuries, such as the menisci and ligaments of the knee.

NOT JUST AN INJURY TO BONE

Injury to the soft tissue is common with high-energy tibial plateau fractures but may also occur with low-energy mechanisms. Ligamentous and musculotendinous soft tissues, which function as the static and dynamic stabilizers of the knee, are at risk when angular, rotational, and axial loads are applied to the lower extremity. In addition, the skin and subcutaneous tissue that surrounds the knee are at significant risk for injury, specifically open fracture.[2,7–10]

In contrast to highly constrained joints such as the hip, the bones provide very little stability to the knee. Therefore, the stability of the knee relies on the surrounding ligaments, capsule, and meniscus. As a result, treatment plans that only focus on the bone alone may not result in the restoration of normal stability and function of the knee.

INCIDENCE OF SOFT TISSUE INJURY ASSOCIATED WITH TIBIAL PLATEAU FRACTURES

In 1994, Bennett and Browner began uncovering the concomitant injuries to the soft tissues associated with tibial plateau fracture. By using a combination of imaging, physical examination, and diagnostic arthroscopy, the incidence of soft tissue injury in 30 patients with tibial plateau fractures was described. They found the overall incidence of soft tissue injury to be 56%, with 20% of patients sustaining injury to the menisci and/or medial collateral ligament (MCL), 10% to the anterior cruciate ligament (ACL), and 3% to the lateral collateral ligament (LCL).[6,11] By applying the Schatzker classification of plateau fractures,[12,13] they also showed a higher rate of soft tissue injury in Schatzker II and Schatzker IV type fractures. More specifically, they noted MCL injury to be most common in type II fractures, whereas meniscal injury was more common in type IV.[6] The high incidence of internal soft tissue derangement was also highlighted in a later article by Colletti and colleagues,[14] in which they reported some form of soft tissue injury in 28 of 29 (97%) acute tibial plateau fractures. Specifically, the incidence of injury to individual structures was as follows: 55% MCL, 45% lateral meniscus, 21% medial meniscus, 34% LCL, 41% ACL, and 28% PCL. However, they

were not able to show a correlation between fracture type or degree of articular depression and the incidence soft tissue injury. Even in minimally displaced tibial plateau fractures that can be treated nonoperatively, it has been shown that complete ligament disruptions and meniscal tears can be present.[15]

In the mid to late 2000s, 2 larger studies really focused on the high incidence of soft tissue injury associated with tibial plateau fractures. In 2005, Gardner and colleagues prospectively performed MRIs on 103 patients with operative tibial plateau fractures. Similar to Colletti's study, 99% of patients had some form of associated injury (Table 1). Injuries to the menisci were the most common soft tissue finding with lateral meniscus pathology being found in 91% of patients. However, the meniscus was not the only soft tissue structure injured. Complete tear or avulsion of at least one ligament was noted in a large percentage of patients (77%). The ACL was the most common ligament injured (57%), followed by LCL, MCL, and PCL, all having similar incidences. Before this study, the other structures of the posterolateral corner (PLC) had not been specifically evaluated. Of the 103 patients, 68% had tears of the popliteofibular ligament, the popliteus tendon, or both.[16]

In 2010, Stannard and colleagues provided what is likely the most comprehensive breakdown of tibial plateau fracture–associated soft tissue injury. They also evaluated 103 tibial plateau fractures with MRI for ligamentous and meniscal injury.[3] Similar to Gardner's findings, 71% of patients had at least one major ligament

Table 1	
Incidence of soft tissue structures injured	
Structure	**% of Cohort (Absolute Number)**
ACL	57% (59)
PCL	28% (29)
MCL	32% (33)
LCL	29% (30)
Medial meniscus	44% (45)
Lateral meniscus	91% (94)
PLC	68% (70)

Data from Gardner MJ, Yacoubian S, Geller D, et al. The incidence of soft tissue injury in operative tibial plateau fractures. A magnetic resonance imaging analysis of 103 patients. *J Orthop Trauma.* 2005;19(2):79-84. https://doi.org/10.1097/00005131-200502000-00002.

group that was torn, whereas 53% tore multiple ligament groups. The overall incidence of meniscus tears was lower in this study (49%) and was equally distributed between the 2 menisci. Also, this paper was the first to show an increasing incidence of ligament injury with the severity of bony injury. Broken down by Schatzker type, they presented the following incidence of ligament injury: type I 46%, type II 45%, type IV 69%, type V 85%, and type VI 79% (Table 2). The authors noted that higher energy fracture types (types IV–VI) had a significantly higher incidence of soft tissue injuries compared with lower energy types (types I–III).[3]

CLINICAL RELEVANCE

Appropriate evaluation and treatment of tibial plateau fractures is an evolving field in its own right. Although there are several well-established treatment paradigms for both bony and ligamentous injuries to the knee, a comprehensive understanding of tibial plateau fracture and associated soft tissue injuries is required to provide maximally effective treatment.

OBSERVATION/ASSESSMENT/INITIAL EVALUATION

Initial assessment of any patient should always begin with a thorough history. Understanding the mechanism of injury can be critical to fully understanding their injury.[2] An axial loading mechanism from a motor vehicle accident may have a different bony and soft tissue injury pattern than an injury sustained during sport. The energy imparted to the soft tissue envelope can help forecast the timing in which definitive surgery can be performed. Therefore,

Table 2	
Incidence of ligament injury by Schatzker type	
Schatzker Type	**% with Ligament Injury**
I	46%
II	45%
IV	69%
V	85%
VI	79%

Note: No Schatzker type III fractures were noted in their study.

Data from Stannard JP, Lopez R, Volgas D. Soft tissue injury of the knee after tibial plateau fractures. *J Knee Surg.* 2010;23(4):187-192. https://doi.org/10.1055/s-0030-1268694.

characterizing the type of injury, either high or low energy, can help decision making.

In regard to physical examination, initial inspection should involve careful evaluation of the patient's soft tissue envelope to assess for open fracture, obvious dislocation or deformity, and general state of the skin, as these factors alone may guide an orthopedist toward potential initial surgical treatment options.[2,7] Thorough assessment of the lower extremity fascial compartments is also critical. Tibial plateau fractures, especially high-energy ones or those associated with a knee dislocation, can lead to compartment syndrome from either continuous metaphyseal hemorrhage into the lower leg or from vascular injury.[2,7,17] Following palpation, there should be a careful assessment of the neurovascular status of the limb with palpation and/or Doppler examination of distal blood flow at the dorsalis pedis and posterior tibial arteries. For high-energy tibial plateau fractures, an ankle brachial index should be obtained.[2] If the value is less than 0.9, the evaluating physician should be immediately suspicious for a vascular injury, and further workup with angiography or vascular surgery consult should be obtained.[2,7,17,18]

Traditional examination of the knee, including range of motion and a ligamentous examination are usually not possible with acute tibial plateau fracture. Oftentimes, advanced imaging and examination under anesthesia are used in lieu of a detailed physical examination of the knee.

IMAGING/ADDITIONAL TESTING

As with most orthopedic injuries, the first diagnostic step after initial assessment is plain radiographs. Standard anteroposterior (AP) and lateral views of the involved knee are required, but the clinician may also obtain oblique views or a modified AP view (beam shoots down the posterior slope of the tibia).[2,7,19] These additional views allow more critical evaluation of the articular surface of the tibial plateau. Radiographs of the contralateral knee may also be beneficial in surgical planning, providing a template for bony reduction.[2] In addition to bony detail, the evaluation of soft tissues also begin with radiographs. Assessment of the medial and lateral joint spaces, joint subluxation in either the coronal or sagittal plane, or disruption of the proximal tibiofibular joint can provide early identification of soft tissue injury. In addition to the tibia, fracture of the fibular head can be a sign of lateral-sided ligamentous injury.

Before the advent of advanced imaging modalities, preoperative stress radiographs were commonly used to identify ligamentous injury.[20] These radiographs have now been replaced with computed tomography (CT) and/or MRI, preoperatively, but stress imaging after fracture stabilization is still routinely used. CT provides excellent detail regarding bony morphology and fracture characteristics, but lacks soft tissue detail.[2,7,13,21] MRI has become the gold standard for use in evaluation of soft tissue injury about the knee; however, its role in the evaluation of patients with tibial plateau fracture remains controversial.[2,3,22] It has been found that current MRI techniques provide excellent bony detail while also providing valuable information regarding the soft tissue. Although we continue to use stress radiographs after fixation to confirm stability, MRI has largely replaced preoperative stress views.

In an effort to replace the need for MRI to identify soft tissue injury, several studies have attempted to correlate fracture characteristics with injury to soft tissue structures of the knee. Gardner and colleagues evaluated 62 patients with Schatzker II tibial plateau fractures. They measured condylar widening and articular depression and used MRI to correlate their findings with the incidence of meniscal pathology. If the patient had greater than 6 mm of lateral articular depression and 5 mm of condylar widening, the lateral meniscus was found to be torn 83% of the time. Injury to the medial meniscus seemed to correlate with greater depression and widening, with 8 mm, instead of 6 mm, seeming to correlate.[23] Similar numbers were found in another study attempting to correlate fracture characteristics with ligamentous injuries. After evaluating 54 patients with tibial plateau fractures, lateral plateau depression greater than or equal to 6 mm or lateral condylar widening greater than or equal to 8 mm were found to be indicators of concomitant cruciate and collateral ligament injuries.[24]

Mui and colleagues compared CT and MRI scans in patients with tibial plateau fractures to assess the accuracy of CT alone in the diagnosis of soft tissue injury. They found that CT scan was 80% sensitive and 98% specific for ligament tear and provided a 98% negative predictive value for individual ligament tears when read by a musculoskeletal-trained radiologist. In their study, although both fracture gap and articular depression were significantly greater in patients with meniscal injury, they could not establish a clear value threshold and concluded that MRI is likely necessary to fully evaluate for meniscal injury.[25] Although a specific amount of depression or condylar widening has yet to be to clearly defined, multiple studies have shown that with increasing depression and condylar widening, the incidence of soft tissue injury also increases.[21,26,27]

Both CT and MRI of tibial plateau fractures have been shown to alter surgical indications and management of these complex injuries.[2,13,28–30] Holt and colleagues[31] found that MRI changed their initial classification in nearly 50% of cases and altered treatment in nearly 20% of cases. Yacoubian and colleagues investigated the interobserver agreement between 3 orthopedic traumatologists for treatment plan and fracture classification based on radiographs, CT, and MRI. They found that fracture classification was agreed on 68% of the time with radiography, 73% with CT, and 85% with MRI. In addition, fracture classification changed 6% of the time with addition of CT and 21% with addition of MRI. There was agreement on management plan 72% of the time with radiography, 77% with radiography and CT, and 86% with radiography and MRI. Overall, MRI altered the treatment plan in 23% of patients.[22] Therefore, compared with CT, MRI seems to alter classification and treatment plans more often.

The role of MRI in evaluation and management of tibial plateau fractures remains controversial, likely due to cost, time, and availability. CT and plain radiographs are cheaper, quicker, and more readily available, however, may not provide the information required to provide ideal care for these complex injuries. In general, there has been little success in establishing reliable radiographic indicators of soft tissue injuries, so many of the investigators recommend MRI for evaluation of at least high-energy, if not all, tibial plateau fractures.[2,3,14,16,22,25,26,31–33] Currently, at our institution, MRI is the advanced imaging modality of choice. Although there is a learning curve for preoperative planning for those who have traditionally used CT, the transition from CT to MRI has been found quite seamless.

THERAPEUTIC OPTIONS/SURGICAL TECHNIQUES

Surgical techniques for external fixation and open reduction and internal fixation (ORIF) of tibial plateau fractures are well established and documented in the literature, with a multitude of approach and implant options based on the fracture characteristics. A foundational principle that is reinforced throughout the literature is that the surgeon must gently and meticulously handle the soft tissues.[2,7] Following the success of staged management of high-energy tibial plafond fractures, Egol and colleagues performed a study on 57 high-energy (Schatzker IV, V, and VI) tibial plateau fractures that received staged management with initial external fixation followed by delayed ORIF or conversion to ring fixator construct. They demonstrated a 5% wound infection rate compared with wound complications of 13% to 88% in prior studies of acute ORIF of similar injuries.[4]

Temporizing external fixation followed by delayed ORIF has become common practice. At our institution, the following treatment paradigm is generally followed. Length-stable, lower-energy, operative tibial plateau fractures with no significant soft tissue envelope disruption undergo MRI scan followed by ORIF acutely. High-energy, length-unstable tibial plateau fractures and/or those associated with significant soft tissue disruption undergo temporizing external fixation, postoperative MRI, followed by delayed ORIF when the soft tissues allow. MRI provides information that not only assists in planning osteosynthesis but also provides the necessary information to plan definitive management of ligamentous and meniscal injury, if present. If the patient is unable to undergo MRI secondary to an incompatible implanted device or other prohibitive issues, CT scan is obtained instead.

Currently, there is very little literature guiding management of soft tissue injuries in combination with tibia plateau fractures. For example, a definitive guide to treatment of a patient with an ACL or MCL tear concomitant with a tibia plateau fracture does not exist. Therefore, most of the way we approach soft tissues is based on experience and the principle of obtaining a stable knee with a good arc of motion.

In general, most lateral approaches to the plateau are performed in conjunction with a submeniscal arthrotomy,[2,7,34,35] and this not only allows for direct visualization of the articular injury for reduction and fixation but also provides an opportunity to evaluate the lateral meniscus and repair it if needed. If preoperative MRI is consistent with PLC injury, the surgical incision is adjusted to allow for access to the fibular head and dissection of the peroneal nerve. In most circumstances, a medial approach for tibial plateau fixation can also be used for repair or reconstruction of the medial ligamentous structures.

In the acute setting, the decision between repair versus reconstruction of collateral ligaments is usually guided by findings on MRI. For mid-substance collateral tears, reconstruction is usually the preferred technique. Repairs are performed for avulsions, commonly off the fibular head for the PLC or off the tibia for the superficial MCL. Also, after fixation of the bony architecture, stress views to evaluate the stability of the knee should always be performed. If coronal plane instability is present, addressing the collaterals is important in management. If collateral instability is recognized later, reconstruction is usually preferred over repair.

Cruciate injuries pose a particularly difficult management problem due to the fact that reconstruction sockets are usually passing through areas of fixation in the tibia. Large, displaced tibial avulsions are usually addressed at the time of ORIF with either screw fixation or suture repair. In many cases, PCL avulsions off the tibia can be repaired using a posteromedial approach to the tibia in conjunction with fixation of the posteromedial plateau fracture fragment. For midsubstance cruciate tears, a staged approach is followed. In this setting, the tibial plateau is repaired via ORIF. Once the bone has adequately healed, the patient is assessed for continued instability associated with either the ACL and/or PCL. If symptoms of instability exist after bony union is achieved, partial removal of implants is performed to facilitate reconstruction. Thankfully, in our experience, this late reconstruction is seldom needed.

Meniscal injuries are addressed by a variety of methods. Usually, lateral meniscus tears are addressed using open techniques through the anterolateral approach to the tibia. If the medial meniscus tear seems significant on MRI, arthroscopy is used at the time of ORIF. Particular attention to the posterior meniscal roots on MRI is important. These injuries can be addressed by open or arthroscopic techniques.

CLINICAL OUTCOMES

There has been very limited correlation between clinical outcomes and specific soft tissue injuries associated with tibial plateau fractures. In 2018, Warner and colleagues evaluated findings on MRI and attempted to correlate those findings with patient outcomes. Interestingly, they were not able to show that soft tissue injury correlated with patient outcomes. However, they did not specifically assess the PLC, which has proved to be a structure vital to knee stability.[36,37] In addition, their incidence of cruciate ligament injury was lower than reported in other studies.[3,16] This could be because the majority (67%) of the fractures included in their study were low-energy (Schatzker I and II) but nonetheless

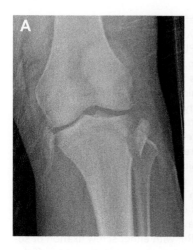
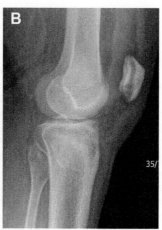

Fig. 1. Plain radiographs of the left knee of a 27-year-old following a motorcycle accident. A depressed lateral plateau fracture is identified with a small fracture of the medial plateau. (*A*) AP view. (*B*) Lateral view.

highlights another inconsistency that needs to be clarified by future studies.[36] In addition, this was a retrospective study and some soft tissue injuries were repaired while others were not. In their treatment algorithm, lateral meniscus tears were repaired at the time of ORIF via submeniscal arthrotomy but medial meniscus tears were not repaired. If there was instability after ORIF, collateral repair was performed but cruciates were not addressed. In addition, this study only included 82 patients, which is severely underpowered to evaluate a causal relationship between specific soft tissue components to outcomes. Although this study was not able to correlate worse clinical outcomes with specific soft tissue injuries, there are some important conclusions that can be made. It does seem that if lateral meniscus tears are addressed at the time of surgery, patients can expect good results. Also, if instability exists after ORIF, soft tissue structures should be addressed. So in essence, this paper solidifies the concept that soft tissue structures cannot be ignored in the management of tibial plateau fractures.

FUTURE DIRECTIONS/GAPS IN LITERATURE

The evaluation and management of soft tissue injuries in patients with tibia plateau fractures continues to evolve. Currently, it is known that many patients have injuries to the ligaments or menisci.[3,4,6,14,16,20–27,31–36,38,39] Although we understand that these injuries exist, we currently do not know if and when we should be addressing them surgically. Further research should evaluate treatment algorithms in a prospective manner to determine which injuries would benefit from repair or reconstruction and which injuries can simply be ignored. Obviously, prospective randomized trials would be ideal, but because of the complicated spectrum of injury, these are quite challenging.

CASE EXAMPLE

A 27-year-old man presented after a motorcycle accident with articular depression and a small fracture of the medial plateau in addition to lateral plateau fracture (Fig. 1). Careful

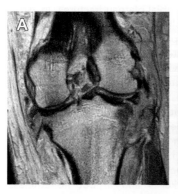
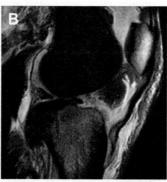

Fig. 2. Representative MRI images demonstrating (*A*) lateral meniscus tear, depressed lateral tibia plateau fracture, MCL disruption, and (*B*) patella tendon avulsion.

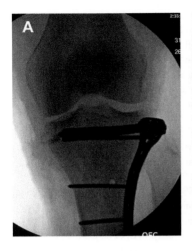
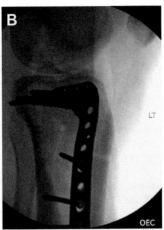

Fig. 3. Fluoroscopic images after ORIF of lateral tibia plateau with repair of the lateral meniscus, repair of the patella tendon, repair of the medial capsule, and repair of the superficial MCL.

evaluation of the MRI scan showed multiple soft tissue injuries, in addition to the plateau fracture. The patient had a peripheral lateral meniscus tear, patella tendon avulsion, tear of the superficial MCL off the tibia, and injury to the deep MCL and capsule (Fig. 2).

A few days after injury, surgical stabilization was performed after edema had resolved. Surgery began with an anterolateral approach to the proximal tibia. The approach included visualization of the patella tendon insertion. A submeniscal arthrotomy was performed, which easily identified the large peripheral lateral meniscus tear and articular depression. Multiple nonabsorbable sutures were placed from outside-in through the capsule and into the meniscus to stabilize the tear. Once the meniscus was repaired, ORIF was performed by elevating the depressed articular surfaces and buttress plating with multiple rafting screws. The patella tendon was repaired back to the tibial tubercle using suture anchors. After stabilization of the lateral plateau and repair of the patella tendon, the patient remained unstable to valgus stress. A medial incision showed complete capsular detachment from the tibia and tearing of the superficial MCL from the tibia. The medial capsule was then repaired to the proximal tibia using suture anchors, and the MCL was also repaired using suture anchors. Final fluoroscopic views are seen in Fig. 3.

SUMMARY

Tibial plateau fractures represent an injury to both bone and soft tissue. Therefore, a multifaceted diagnostic and therapeutic approach should be followed. MRI should be considered as a replacement to CT to better evaluate both the bony and soft tissue injuries. Although specific treatment algorithms for all of the soft tissue injuries are not currently available, the general concept of restoring stability and repair of lateral meniscus injuries seems to be appropriate at this time.

CLINICS CARE POINTS

1. Tibial plateau fractures should not be thought of as only a bony injury. An appropriate treatment approach should take into account the soft tissues in addition to the fracture.
2. Suspicion for soft tissue derangement should accompany any tibial plateau fracture, but increasing energy, fracture displacement, and/or articular depression should heighten that suspicion.
3. In order to diagnose and plan for management of the entire injury, MRI should be considered as a routine replacement of CT.
4. Lateral meniscus tears should be repaired if diagnosed at the time of ORIF or by preoperative MRI.
5. The goal of treatment should be to provide a stable knee through a normal range of motion. Many times this is accomplished by ORIF alone, but the surgeon should be prepared to repair or reconstruct collaterals if needed.

DISCLOSURE

Dr J.D. Adams is a paid consultant of Arthrex. He is also committee member for the AAOS and teaching faculty for AO North America. Dr M.F. Loeffler has nothing to disclose.

REFERENCES

1. Elsoe R, Larsen P, Nielsen NPH, et al. Population-based epidemiology of tibial plateau fractures. Orthopedics 2015;38(9):e780–6.

2. Browner B, Jupiter J, Christian K, et al. Skeletal trauma: basic science, management, and reconstruction. 6th edition. Philadelphia: Elsevier Inc.; 2019.

3. Stannard JP, Lopez R, Volgas D. Soft tissue injury of the knee after tibial plateau fractures. J Knee Surg 2010;23(4):187–92.

4. Tejwani NC, Achan P. Staged management of high-energy proximal tibia fractures. Bull Hosp Jt Dis 2004;62(1-2):62–6.

5. Watson JT. High-energy fractures of the tibial plateau. Orthop Clin North Am 1994;25(4):723–52. Available at: http://www.ncbi.nlm.nih.gov/pubmed/8090483. Accessed January 24, 2020.

6. Bennett WF, Browner B. Tibial plateau fractures: A study of associated soft tissue injuries. J Orthop Trauma 1994;8(3):183–8.

7. Wiesel SW, Parvizi J, Rothman RH, et al. Operative techniques in orthopaedic surgery. 2nd edition. Philadelphia, PA: Wolters Kluwer; 2016.

8. Prat-Fabregat S, Camacho-Carrasco P. Treatment strategy for tibial plateau fractures: An update. EFORT Open Rev 2016;1(5):225–32.

9. Giordano CP, Koval KJ, Zuckerman JD, et al. Fracture blisters. Clin Orthop Relat Res 1994;(307):214–21.

10. Berkson EM, Virkus WW. High-energy tibial plateau fractures. J Am Acad Orthop Surg 2006;14(1):20–31.

11. Ibrahim DA, Swenson A, Sassoon A, et al. Classifications In Brief: The Tscherne Classification of Soft Tissue Injury. Clin Orthop Relat Res 2017;475(2):560–4.

12. Schatzker J, McBroom R. The tibial plateau fracture. The Toronto experience 1968-1975. Clin Orthop Relat Res 1979;(138):94–104.

13. Markhardt BK, Gross JM, Monu JUV. Schatzker classification of tibial plateau fractures: Use of CT and MR imaging improves assessment. Radiographics 2009;29(2):585–97.

14. Colletti P, Greenberg H, Terk MR. MR findings in patients with acute tibial plateau fractures. Comput Med Imaging Graph 1996;20(5):389–94.

15. Shepherd L, Abdollahi K, Lee J, et al. The prevalence of soft tissue injuries in nonoperative tibial plateau fractures as determined by magnetic resonance imaging. J Orthop Trauma 2002;16(9):628–31.

16. Gardner MJ, Yacoubian S, Geller D, et al. The incidence of soft tissue injury in operative tibial plateau fractures. A magnetic resonance imaging analysis of 103 patients. J Orthop Trauma 2005;19(2):79–84.

17. Rihn JA, Groff YJ, Harner CD, et al. The acutely dislocated knee: evaluation and management. J Am Acad Orthop Surg 2004;12(5):334–46.

18. Mills WJ, Barei DP, McNair P. The value of the ankle-brachial index for diagnosing arterial injury after knee dislocation: A prospective study. J Trauma 2004;56(6):1261–5.

19. Moore TM, Harvey JP. Roentgenographic measurement of tibial plateau depression due to fracture. J Bone Joint Surg Am 1974;56(1):155–60.

20. Delamarter RB, Hohl M, Hopp E. Ligament injuries associated with tibial plateau fractures. Clin Orthop Relat Res 1990;(250):226–33.

21. Tang HC, Chen IJ, Yeh YC, et al. Correlation of parameters on preoperative CT images with intra-articular soft-tissue injuries in acute tibial plateau fractures: A review of 132 patients receiving ARIF. Injury 2017;48(3):745–50.

22. Yacoubian SV, Nevins RT, Sallis JG, et al. Impact of MRI on treatment plan and fracture classification of tibial plateau fractures. J Orthop Trauma 2002;16(9):632–7.

23. Gardner MJ, Yacoubian S, Geller D, et al. Prediction of soft-tissue injuries in Schatzker II tibial plateau fractures based on measurements of plain radiographs. J Trauma 2006;60(2):319–24.

24. Wang J, Wei J, Wang M. The distinct prediction standards for radiological assessments associated with soft tissue injuries in the acute tibial plateau fracture. Eur J Orthop Surg Traumatol 2015;25(5):913–20.

25. Mui LW, Engelsohn E, Umans H. Comparison of CT and MRI in patients with tibial plateau fracture: Can CT findings predict ligament tear or meniscal injury? Skeletal Radiol 2007;36(2):145–51.

26. Spiro AS, Regier M, de Oliveira AN, et al. The degree of articular depression as a predictor of soft-tissue injuries in tibial plateau fracture. Knee Surg Sports Traumatol Arthrosc 2013;21(3):564–70.

27. Chang H, Zheng Z, Shao D, et al. Incidence and radiological predictors of concomitant meniscal and cruciate ligament injuries in operative tibial plateau fractures: a prospective diagnostic study. Sci Rep 2018;8(1):1–9.

28. Chan PSH, Klimkiewicz JJ, Luchetti WT, et al. Impact of CT scan on treatment plan and fracture classification of tibial plateau fractures. J Orthop Trauma 1997;11(7):484–9.

29. Macarini L, Murrone M, Marini S, et al. Tibial plateau fractures: evaluation with multidetector-CT. Radiol Med 2004;108(5-6):503–14. Available at: http://www.ncbi.nlm.nih.gov/pubmed/15722996. Accessed March 11, 2020.

30. Van den Berg J, Struelens B, Nijs S, et al. Value of three-dimensional computed tomography

reconstruction in the treatment of posterior tibial plateau fractures. Knee 2020. https://doi.org/10.1016/j.knee.2019.11.001.

31. Holt MD, Williams LA, Dent CM. MRI in the management of tibial plateau fractures. Injury 1995; 26(9):595–9.

32. Lee SY, Jee WH, Jung JY, et al. Lateral meniscocapsular separation in patients with tibial plateau fractures: Detection with magnetic resonance imaging. J Comput Assist Tomogr 2015;39(2):257–62.

33. Kolb JP, Regier M, Vettorazzi E, et al. Prediction of meniscal and ligamentous injuries in lateral tibial plateau fractures based on measurements of lateral plateau widening on multidetector computed tomography scans. Biomed Res Int 2018;2018. https://doi.org/10.1155/2018/5353820.

34. Stahl D, Serrano-Riera R, Collin K, et al. Operatively treated meniscal tears associated with tibial plateau fractures: A report on 661 patients. J Orthop Trauma 2015;29(7):322–4.

35. Tekin AÇ, Çakar M, Esenyel CZ, et al. An evaluation of meniscus tears in lateral tibial plateau fractures and repair results. J Back Musculoskelet Rehabil 2016;29(4):845–51.

36. Warner SJ, Garner MR, Schottel PC, et al. The effect of soft tissue injuries on clinical outcomes after tibial plateau fracture fixation. J Orthop Trauma 2018;32(3):141–7.

37. Stannard JP, Stannard JT, Cook JL. Repair or reconstruction in acute posterolateral instability of the knee: decision making and surgical technique introduction. J Knee Surg 2015;28(6):450–4.

38. Porrino J, Richardson ML, Hovis K, et al. Association of tibial plateau fracture morphology with ligament disruption in the context of multiligament knee injury. Curr Probl Diagn Radiol 2018;47(6): 410–6.

39. Park H-J, Lee H-D, Cho JH. The efficacy of meniscal treatment associated with lateral tibial plateau fractures. Knee Surg Relat Res 2017;29(2):137–43.

Pediatrics

Traumatic Patellar Dislocations in Childhood and Adolescents

Nathan L. Grimm, MD[a,b,*], Benjamin J. Levy, MD[b],
Andrew E. Jimenez, MD[b], Allison E. Crepeau, MD[b,c],
James Lee Pace, MD[c,d,e]

KEYWORDS

• Patella • Patellofemoral • Instability • Subluxation • Dislocation • Knee • Injury

KEY POINTS

- Patellar instability is a common problem in young patients, which can be the result of a single or recurrent traumatic event and typically is due to one or a combination of anatomic aberrancies.
- Early recognition through appropriate history and physical examination can help prevent future events and reduce the risk of associated injuries.
- Awareness of associated injuries with patellar dislocation and appropriate imaging will help guide the surgeon's treatment.
- Surgical treatment can range from minimally invasive all arthroscopic treatment to open ligament reconstruction, tibial tubercle osteotomy, and trochleoplasty.
- Both operative and nonoperative treatments benefit from rehabilitation in patients who have sustained patellar dislocations.

INTRODUCTION

Lateral patellar instability is a common problem in the pediatric and adolescent population. It is one of the most frequent acute knee injuries in this age group, with an annual incidence that has been estimated between 23.2 and 43 per 100,000.[1–3] Further, one population-based study reported that 75% of all first-time patellar dislocations occurred in patients aged 25 years or younger.[4] Multiple studies have suggested that women are at higher risk than men for patellar instability.[2,5] Seventy percent of first-time patellar dislocations occurred while doing sporting activities or dance.[2,6] Indirect or noncontact injuries account for 59% of first-time patellar dislocations.[5]

The overall risk of recurrence after a first-time patellar dislocation in patients aged 18 years and younger is around 34% to 38%.[5,6] However, multiple risk factors have been identified that increase the risk of recurrence. These include trochlear dysplasia, skeletal immaturity, history of contralateral dislocation, patella alta, and participation in sports.[5–7] The combination of multiple risk factors can bring the recurrence rate up to 88%.[5]

Development of symptomatic patellofemoral arthritis is the primary long-term concern following lateral patellar dislocation. Cumulative incidence has been shown to be as high as 39% to 49% at 25 years. This is compared with a matched cohort without patellar instability, which had a patellofemoral arthritis rate of 8% at 25 years.[4] Development of arthritis is most strongly correlated with osteochondral injury at the time of dislocation, but other risk factors include female sex, younger age at primary

[a] Idaho Sports Medicine Institute, 1188 West University Drive, Boise, ID 83701, USA; [b] Division of Sports Medicine, UConn Health, 120 Dowling Way, Farmington, CT 06032, USA; [c] Elite Sports Medicine at Connecticut Children's, 282 Washington Street, Hartford, CT 06106, USA; [d] UConn Health, Division of Sports Medicine, Department of Orthopedics, 120 Dowling Way, Farmington, CT 06032, USA; [e] Hamden, CT, USA
* Corresponding author. UConn Health, Division of Sports Medicine, 120 Dowling Way, Farmington, CT 06032.
E-mail address: N8grimm@gmail.com

Orthop Clin N Am 51 (2020) 481–491
https://doi.org/10.1016/j.ocl.2020.06.005
0030-5898/20/© 2020 Elsevier Inc. All rights reserved.

dislocation, recurrent dislocation, and trochlear dysplasia.[1,4]

ANATOMY AND BIOMECHANICS

The patellofemoral joint is arguably one of the most dynamically complex joints in the body. The 3 osseous structures that provide the skeletal support include the femur, tibia, and patella. Structural abnormalities of 1, 2, or all 3 of these bones can have serious effects on the function and stability of the patellofemoral joint.[8]

A dysplastic trochlear groove has been shown to be the most common anatomic risk factor for patellar dislocation.[5,6,8–12] After approximately 30° of flexion the trochlear groove is the principle static patellar restraint.[8] However, in patients with trochlear dysplasia the proximal aspect of this track can be shallow, flat, or even convex, which diminishes or obliterates the osseous restraint normally provided.[13,14]

The most widely accepted metric to define trochlear dysplasia is a sulcus angle of greater than 145° as measured, preferably, on an axial computed tomographic (CT) scan or MRI study.[15]

Abnormal patellar height, referred to as patella alta, also plays a significant role in patellar instability.[13] Several measurements have been devised to calculate and define patella alta[16–22] and are discussed later.

A lateralized tibial tubercle has been associated with patellar instability.[23] The tibial tubercle to trochlear groove (TT-TG) is a known measure of patellar instability.[24] Although there is variability among what is considered pathologic, a TT-TG is typically considered pathologic when measured greater than 20 mm.[15] However, in children this value may differ with age, and percentile-based growth charts have been developed to help normalize this value.[25] More recent studies have called into question how often the tibial tubercle is truly located in a pathologically lateral position or if it is secondary to rotation of the tibia.[26,27]

Although more rare, axial plane malalignment at the femur in the form of femoral anteversion or coronal plane malalignment in the form of genu valgum can create a lever arm that increases the force seen on the patella, increasing the lateral pull and predisposing to dislocation and lateral patellofemoral overload.[23]

On the lateral side of the knee, static soft tissue stabilizers are characterized by the complex layer of tissue collectively called the lateral retinaculum. Increased tension on the lateral retinaculum can increase the lateral patellar tilt, overload the lateral facet of the patellofemoral joint, and contribute to patellar instability. In contrast, on the medial side of the knee, the medial patellofemoral complex (MPFC)[28] and more specifically the medial patellofemoral ligament (MPFL) is the principle soft tissue restraint to lateral patellar translation. The primary function of this structure is to provide a static restraint in the first 30° of knee flexion before engagement of the patella in the trochlea. Although the ligament is relatively thin it can tolerate loads of up to 200N before failure.[29]

CLINICAL HISTORY AND PHYSICAL EXAMINATION

A comprehensive history is a critical starting point in the evaluation of any patient with patellar instability.[30] Any previous knee symptoms, surgeries, or diagnoses should be noted. Not uncommonly, the patient will experience anterior knee pain, apprehension, or a feeling of giving way before the onset of dislocation events.

A complete musculoskeletal examination should follow the history. This includes noting and investigating any features of skeletal dysplasia, joint hypermobility, or syndromic features.[31] Coronal and axial plane alignment of the lower extremities should be assessed. A focused examination on the affected knee includes range of motion, points of tenderness, and ligamentous testing. Patellar height, crepitus on active range of motion, tracking, translation, and the presence of apprehension should be carefully evaluated and can be used to gauge the severity of instability. Increased patellar translation and apprehension to lateral translation of the patella are classic physical examination findings in patella instability. Although this is typically done with the affected knee in full extension, checking lateral translation and apprehension with the knee in increasing levels of knee flexion can give the examiner insights into the degree of trochlear dysplasia and/or patella alta. Most patellae will engage in a normally shaped trochlea around 30° to 40° of knee flexion. At this point, patellar translation should be at a minimum. If the patient continues to experience increased translation and/or apprehension beyond this amount of knee flexion, trochlear dysplasia and/or patella alta is suspected. Abnormalities detected on physical examination should be carefully scrutinized and further evaluated with imaging.[32]

IMAGING

Initial imaging of patients presenting with complaints of patellofemoral instability in the clinic should include a standard series of radiographs, including weight-bearing anteroposterior (AP), weight-bearing 45° posteroanterior (PA) flexion, lateral, and axial views. The Dejour classification is the most recognized tool for qualifying and characterizing trochlear dysplasia[33] (**Fig. 1**). In addition, assessment of patellar height is possible using a lateral radiograph. Numerous methods of measurement have been described for this, including Insall-Salvati, Blackburne-Peel, and Caton-Deschamps (CD) ratios.[34] The authors of this article prefer an MRI-based evaluation of patellar height.

Although there is added radiation exposure, there is utility for CT scans due to superior bony visualization. Axial evaluation of dysplasia and TT-TG measurement can be performed. Given the utility of MRI to perform similar evaluations while avoiding radiation exposure, CT currently is reserved for evaluation of rotational alignment[34] (**Fig. 2**).

MRI is invariably recommended for evaluation and treatment determination. MRI allows for an acute evaluation for osteochondral injuries[35] as well as overall evaluation of chondral surfaces. MRI also shows integrity of soft tissue restraints,

namely the MPFL.[36] Assessments typically made on radiographs can be made on MRI with superior accuracy.[37,38] MRI also allows for quantitative analysis of trochlear dysplasia including the lateral trochlear inclination (LTI) angle (**Fig. 3**), a measurement shown to be more reliable and perhaps more direct than the Dejour classification.[39] MRI is also a reliable way to evaluate patellar height. Most previously mentioned measures of patella alta are commonly evaluated via sagittal MRI images.[40] In addition, the patellotrochlear index (PTI) can be evaluated on MRI. The PTI is a measure of patellar and trochlear chondral overlap and may be a more functional representation of patellar height[16] (**Fig. 4**).

TREATMENT—NONSURGICAL

There was 100% agreement within the surgeons of the International Patellofemoral Study Group (IPSG) that a first-time patellar dislocation, in the absence of an operative osteochondral fracture or lesion requiring excision or repair, should be treated nonoperatively.[41] In the absence of spontaneous reduction, treatment of acute patella dislocations involves initial closed reduction achieved with extension of the knee combined with gentle medially directed force of the patella. Supportive bracing involves a patellar stabilization brace that has a lateral buttress. Immediate weight-bearing with crutch assistance for comfort and balance is initiated along with full range of motion. The patellar stabilization brace is typically worn for 6 weeks to allow the medial retinacular tissues to heal. Compressive dressings as well as ice should be used to reduce swelling and aid with restoration of quadriceps function.[30,42] There should be a low threshold for ordering an MRI after a traumatic patellar dislocation, as the risk of osteochondral injury in adolescent patients may be as high as 50%.[43,44]

If a screening MRI is negative and the decision is made to proceed with conservative management, a referral to formal physical therapy is made. Early rehabilitation focuses on closed chain exercises and nonimpact endurance. Impact activities may be initiated as early as 6 weeks after injury if the patient has regained full motion, has resolution of the effusion, and has demonstrated appropriate strength gains. However, some patients may take significantly longer. Athletic activity can be resumed once strength has returned to at least 80% of normal and sport-specific agility has been regained or 2 to 3 months has passed and the patient does not demonstrate any signs of residual patellar

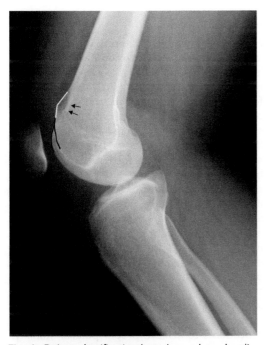

Fig. 1. Dejour classification based on a lateral radiograph. There are 3 signs: the crossing sign (*black line*), supratrochlear spur (*yellow line*), and double contour sign (*black arrows*). Dejour A shows only the crossing sign. Dejour B shows the crossing sign and a supratrochlear spur. Dejour C has a crossing sign and a double contour sign and Dejour D has all 3 signs.

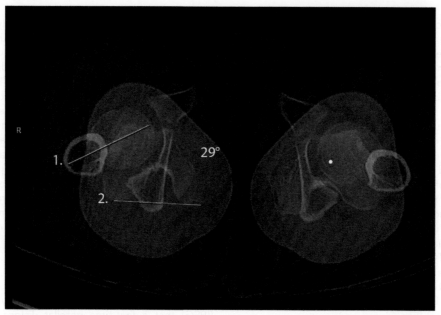

Fig. 2. Rotational profile CT scan. Measurement is made between a line connecting the center of the femoral head and the midportion of the femoral shaft at the level of the lesser trochanter and the posterior femoral condyles. In this example, femoral anteversion is 29°.

apprehension on examination. Garth and Pomphrey reported on return to full activity in 68% of their conservatively treated patients between 3 and 8 weeks.[45] Commonly, a patella stabilizing brace can be used for the first 2 to 3 months after return to athletics. McConnel taping or patella stabilizing braces may serve to help with proprioceptive function but there is no literature to suggest that they reduce the rates of redislocation.[30,42]

Recurrent subluxation and dislocation rates after nonoperative treatment can be as high as 50% to 85%.[5,43,46] The current literature on this is limited with significant variability in patient population and treatment methodologies. Often times the decision to proceed with nonoperative versus operative treatment depends on taking the individual patient and their corresponding history, risk factors, activity level, and expectations into consideration.[30,47]

TREATMENT—SURGICAL

Given the relatively high rate of recurrent instability with conservative management, many patients ultimately require surgical intervention. The most important step in deciding on what surgical procedure to perform on a patient with patellar instability is identifying the underlying reason for the instability. As described earlier, it is of paramount importance to perform a thorough history, complete clinical examination from hip to ankle, and obtain relevant

imaging based off of your findings. These steps are not only for accurate diagnosis bute also for surgical planning.

Patellar Tilt

For the management of lateral patellar tilt due to lateral tightness and opposing medial laxity, an isolated lateral retinacular release (LRR) or lateral retinacular lengthening (LRL) can be performed.[48] With current arthroscopic technology, the LRR is typically done arthroscopically.[48] In comparison, the LRL must be done open (**Fig. 5**). However, proponents argue that LRL is more precise and avoids the risk of medial instability.[48] Furthermore, this is the preferred technique by most of the surgeons within the IPSG.[49] Of importance, however, the consensus agreement among members of the IPSG is that an isolated lateral release or lengthening is never appropriate for the treatment of patellar instability.[41] Given that patellar tilt, in the setting of patellar instability, represents an abnormal state of medial retinacular incompetence and lateral retinacular tightness, an LRR or LRL should be performed in conjunction with other procedures to achieve proper patellar stability. There are no current recommendations as to when patellar tilt should be treated as part of an overall surgical plan. Thus, it must be up to the judgment of the treating surgeon. The senior author, who is a member of IPSG, performs an LRL as part of a comprehensive soft tissue

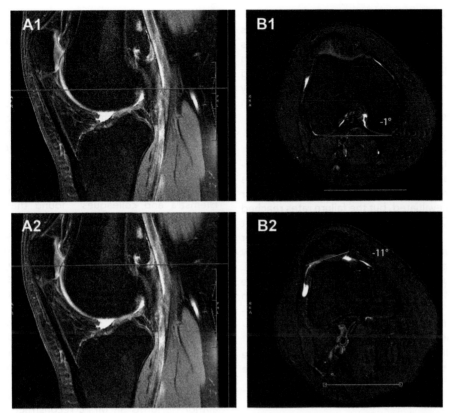

Fig. 3. Two image LTI measurement technique. (A1 & A2) Using a sagittal MRI as a cross reference, the most proximal aspect of the trochlear cartilage is identified on an axial MRI. The angle of the lateral cartilaginous surface is made relative to a horizontal line using the Cobb angle function on the imaging software. In this example, the proximal trochlea is convex so a best fit line is drawn from the lateral trochlea through the apex of the convexity. A convex trochlea will be given a negative value as the angle is obtuse towards the medial aspect of the knee. A normally shaped trochlea would have an inclination angle that would be acute towards the medial aspect of the knee. In this example, the measurement is −11°. (B1 & B2) A second angular measure is taken further distal where the posterior femoral condyles are well formed. Using the Cobb angle function again, this angle is formed between the condyles and a horizontal line again. The condyles are externally rotated 1° so again, the angle is obtuse relative to the medial aspect of the knee and is assigned a value of -1°. The LTI is calculated by subtracting the condyle measurement from the proximal trochlear measurement: −11° to (−1°) = −10°.

retensioning for virtually every patellar stabilization case.

Patella Alta

There are 2 commonly used options to correct patellar height in patients with pathologic patella alta. The first is a distalization of the patellar tendon attachment with a tibial tubercle osteotomy. The second is a plication of the patellar tendon. The first, and perhaps more common, procedure of the 2 options has many advantages. This procedure not only allows for normalizing the patellar position in the sagittal plane but also allows for correcting coronal plane deformity, typically through a medialization.[50] However, this technique carries risks of nonunion, fracture, and loss of fixation,[51] but this may not be an option in the skeletally

immature athlete given the open tubercle apophysis. However, an all-soft-tissue procedure of shortening the patellar tendon has been described[52] for skeletally immature patients. Unfortunately, at the time of this writing, there are no reports to support this technique outside of the cerebral palsy literature.

Prior publications have suggested that a CD ratio greater than 1.2 to 1.4 represents pathologic alta that could be corrected.[50,53,54] However, these represent small case series or systematic reviews of small case series. Although the results reported have been favorable, larger comparative studies are needed to help define a firmer indication for distalization. The senior author currently prefers to use the PTI. If the PTI is less than 20% and there are no other identifiable pathologic processes then a distalization procedure is considered. If the PTI is less than 10% and there are other pathologies present, correction of both is considered. Given the incidence of complications with distalizing the osteotomies,[51] the senior author currently prefers the patellar tendon imbrication technique.

Torn Medial Patellofemoral Ligament

MPFL injury is ubiquitous with traumatic dislocations,[55] and MPFL incompetence is universal is the setting of recurrent instability. MPFL repair has been evaluated, but the failure rates reached almost 30%.[56] This failure is likely due to the fact that the MPFL repair does not address or compensate for underlying pathoanatomy (dysplasia, alta, etc.). Comparatively, MPFL reconstruction increases the strength of the native MPFL by augmentation with a tendon graft,[57,58] which compensates for any pathoanatomy. MPFL reconstruction has shown equivalent results with both autograft and allograft.[59] Thus, MPFL reconstruction has become the gold standard for medial soft tissue stability.[57,58,60,61]

Of technical importance is the location of the reconstruction on the femoral side as described by Schottle and colleagues.[62] In the skeletally immature patient, this point has been shown to be distal to the femoral physis.[63] Final graft tension is typically set between 30° and 60° of knee flexion.[57,58,64] Other variations of MPFL reconstruction exist, such as medial quadriceps tendon femoral ligament reconstruction.[65,66] However, there are no comparative studies between these techniques.

It should be noted that MPFL reconstruction is compensatory surgery that has its limitations. Hiemstra and colleagues[67] found that higher levels of trochlear dysplasia were directly correlated to lower patient-reported outcomes when MPFL reconstruction was performed in isolation. A recent Danish registry study found that 21% of patients after MPFL reconstruction had either recurrent instability or persistent pain at 8 years. This rate was 29% in patients aged 10 to 17 years.[68] A systematic review also found that patients with trochlear dysplasia who underwent MPFL reconstruction in isolation versus those who had a trochleoplasty in combination with soft tissue rebalancing had a lower risk of repeat instability.[69] In general, the senior author performs an MPFL reconstruction combined with an LRL in isolation for patients with mild to moderate underlying pathoanatomy. For patients with high-grade pathoanatomy, the MPFL reconstruction and LRL are performed in combination with a procedure to treat the underlying problem.

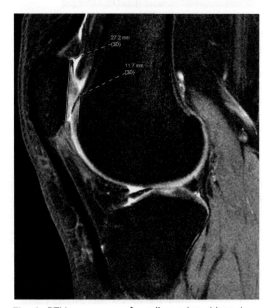

Fig. 4. PTI is a measure of patellar and trochlear chondral overlap. The sagittal MRI image with the longest proximal to distal view of the patella is selected. The length of the cartilaginous patella is measured as is the length of the trochlea that is in contact with the cartilaginous patella. The trochlear length is divided by the patellar length. If the preference is to express this as a percentage, it is multiplied by 100. In this example, the PTI is 11.7/27.2 = 0.43. 0.43 × 100 = 43%.

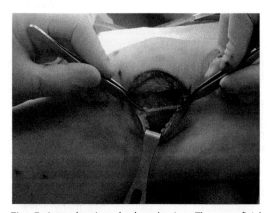

Fig. 5. Lateral retinacular lengthening. The superficial layer of the retinaculum is sharply elevated of the lateral patella and the interval between the superficial and deep is dissected. The deep layer is elevated off the lateral distal femur at a more posterior location. At the end of the procedure, the knee is flexed 70°, and the superficial layer is brought back to the deep layer and it is sewed in place at whatever position it comfortably lies.

Increased Tibial Tubercle to Trochlear Groove Distance

In the setting of an increased TT-TG distance, distal realignment with an anteromedialization (AMZ) producing tibial tubercle osteotomy (TTO) has been the preferred technique by US surgeons.[41] First described by John Fulkerson,[70] the technique allows for off-loading of the patellofemoral cartilage and medializing the lateral force vector on the patella.[71] Although long-term outcomes on TTO alone are good, more recent literature supports adding an MPFL reconstruction to lower redislocation rates.[72] In skeletally immature patients, the Roux-Goldthwait procedure or medial patellar tendon transfer has been described.[73–75] These options can spare the tibial tubercle apophysis but the clinical reports are sparse. Given that recent literature suggests that an increased TT-TG may be due more to dynamic external tibial rotation, accepted surgical indications for distal realignment have been called into question.[26,27,76]

Trochlear Dysplasia

Although trochleoplasty (Fig. 6) has been performed for many years in Europe, it has been slow to be accepted in the United States. Nonetheless, most of the IPSG members agree there is a role for trochleoplasty.[41] The indications for performing a trochleoplasty are controversial. There is consensus that "high-grade" dysplasia is a reasonable indication, but what constitutes high grade is still debated.[13,77–82] A recent consensus statement from a joint workshop sponsored by the American Orthopedic Society for Sports Medicine and Patellofemoral Foundation recommended trochleoplasty in the setting of a J-sign on physical examination, a supratrochlear spur greater than or equal to 5 mm and a convex proximal trochlea.[76]

Despite a disagreement on indications, there are several reports with short- and long-term outcomes after trochleoplasty, showing very reliable outcomes with regard to stability and patient satisfaction.[77–80,82–88] One systematic review comparing trochleoplasty to MPFL reconstruction for patellar instability found no significant difference in redislocation.[89] However, the degree of dysplasia was not evaluated so it is difficult to draw conclusions. Conversely, another systematic review found superior rates of postoperative stability and a trend toward less arthritic progression when trochleoplasty was compared with nontrochleoplasty procedures in patients with severe trochlear dysplasia.[90] A third systematic review, looking exclusively at patients who underwent trochleoplasty found reliable patient outcomes, low redislocation rates, and low complication rates after trohcleoplasty.[83] Regarding skeletal immaturity, a recent report by Nelitz and colleagues[91] showed that a thin-flap trochleoplasty performed at or within 2 years of growth remaining did not result in any growth disturbance at the distal femoral physis.

Given the strong association between trochlear dysplasia and chondral defects/progressive arthritis,[92–95] good chondrocyte viability after trochleoplasty,[96] improved patellofemoral congruence after trochleoplasty,[77,97] and the abovementioned clinical results, a trochleoplasty

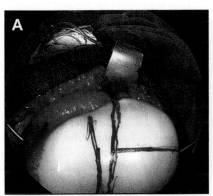 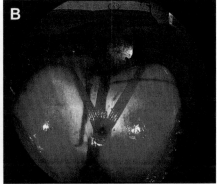

Fig. 6. Groove deepening trochleoplasty. (A) Before trochleoplasty. There is a severely dysplastic trochlea with a very prominent central trochlear prominence/spur. There are 3 purple lines. The most medial purple line is in the native and pathologically medial, trochlear groove. The second, slightly more lateral line is where the new, more lateral, trochlear groove will be placed. This is almost always directly in the center of the convexity/spur. The third lateral and horizontal line represents a demarcation between dysplastic proximal trochlea and more distal, normal trochlea. (B) After trochleoplasty. A central knotless suture anchor holds several strands of #1 Vicryl in place that are then brought proximal and help in place with more suture anchors to hold the thin osteochondral flap in place.

represents an attractive option for patients with patellar instability due to high-grade trochlear dysplasia. The senior author will typically indicate a patient for a trochleoplasty (in combination with soft tissue retensioning via MPFL reconstruction and LRL) when the proximal trochlea is flat or convex. Quantification of dysplasia is via the LTI angle.[39] When the LTI is 0° (flat) or negative (convex), a trochleoplasty is indicated. At this time, however, this is a level V recommendation.

SUMMARY

The patellofemoral joint is dynamic and complex. A patellar dislocation can present significant pain, morbidity, and loss of activity for a young person. In addition, associated osteochondral injuries can add challenge to the treatment of this injury. Of paramount importance is identifying the underlying problem that caused the patella to dislocate via history, physical examination, and imaging. Conservative management is a reasonable start for first-time dislocators without an acute osteochondral fracture, but many patients will ultimately require surgical intervention. Surgical intervention should be tailored to either compensate for (mild pathoanatomy) or treat (severe pathoanatomy) the underlying problem and attention needs to be paid to the open physis in the setting of skeletal immaturity. A detailed understanding of the surgical anatomy and biomechanics will help the treating surgeon achieve the most favorable outcome for the patient with patellar instability.

CLINICS CARE POINTS

- Clinical exam should always include evaluation for femoral anteversion to rule out axial plane malalignment.
- If a large effusion is present, it is important to obtain an MRI to rule-out osteochondral fractures, which can easily be missed.
- Lateral trochlear inclination angle (LTI), as measured on MRI, is a valuable measurement to assess for trochlear dysplasia.
- A laterally-based incision is a utilitarian approach for patellar instability surgery as it allows for a lateral lengthening and trochleoplasty while still being able to access the medial patella for MPFL fixation through a single incision.

DISCLOSURE

Dr J. Lee Pace is a paid consultant for Arthrex, Inc. receiving both consulting fees and research funding. All other authors have nothing to disclose.

REFERENCES

1. Sanders TL, Pareek A, Hewett TE, et al. Incidence of first-time lateral patellar dislocation: a 21-year population-based study. Sports Health 2018;10(2):146–51.
2. Fithian DC, Paxton EW, Stone ML, et al. Epidemiology and natural history of acute patellar dislocation. Am J Sports Med 2004;32(5):1114–21.
3. Nietosvaara Y, Aalto K, Kallio P. Acute patellar dislocation in children: incidence and associated osteochondral fractures. J Pediatr Orthop 1994; 14:513–5.
4. Sanders TL, Pareek A, Johnson NR, et al. Patellofemoral arthritis after lateral patellar dislocation: a matched population-based analysis. Am J Sports Med 2017;45(5):1012–7.
5. Jaquith BP, Parikh SN. Predictors of recurrent patellar instability in children and adolescents after first-time dislocation. J Pediatr Orthop 2017;37(7):484–90.
6. Lewallen LW, McIntosh AL, Dahm DL. Predictors of recurrent instability after acute patellofemoral dislocation in pediatric and adolescent patients. Am J Sports Med 2013;41(3):575–81.
7. Lewallen L, McIntosh A, Dahm D. First-time patellofemoral dislocation: risk factors for recurrent instability. J Knee Surg 2015;28(4):303–9.
8. Bollier M, Fulkerson JP. The role of trochlear dysplasia in patellofemoral instability. J Am Acad Orthop Surg 2011;19(1):8–16.
9. Parikh SN, Lykissas MG, Gkiatas I. Predicting risk of recurrent patellar dislocation. Curr Rev Musculoskelet Med 2018;11(2):253–60.
10. Arendt EA, Askenberger M, Agel J, et al. Risk of redislocation after primary patellar dislocation: a clinical prediction model based on magnetic resonance imaging variables. Am J Sports Med 2018; 46(14):3385–90.
11. Sanders TL, Pareek A, Hewett TE, et al. High rate of recurrent patellar dislocation in skeletally immature patients: a long-term population-based study. Knee Surg Sports Traumatol Arthrosc 2017;26(4):1037–43.
12. Christensen TC, Sanders TL, Pareek A, et al. Risk factors and time to recurrent ipsilateral and contralateral patellar dislocations. Am J Sports Med 2017; 45(9):2105–10.
13. Dejour D, Le Coultre B. Osteotomies in patellofemoral instabilities. Sports Med Arthrosc Rev 2007;15(1):39–46.
14. Van Haver A, De Roo K, De Beule M, et al. The effect of trochlear dysplasia on patellofemoral biomechanics: a cadaveric study with simulated

trochlear deformities. Am J Sports Med 2015;43(6): 1354–61.

15. Dejour H, Walch G, Nove-Josserand L, et al. Factors of patellar instability: an anatomic radiographic study. Knee Surg Sports Traumatol Arthrosc 1994;2(1):19–26.

16. Biedert RM, Albrecht S. The patellotrochlear index: a new index for assessing patellar height. Knee Surg Sports Traumatol Arthrosc 2006;14(8):707–12.

17. Blackburne JS, Peel TE. A new method of measuring patellar height. J Bone Joint Surg Br 1977;59(2):241–2.

18. Caton J, Deschamps G, Chambat P, et al. [Patella infera. Apropos of 128 cases]. Rev Chir Orthop Reparatrice Appar Mot 1982;68(5):317–25.

19. de Carvalho A, Holst Andersen A, Topp S, et al. A method for assessing the height of the patella. Int Orthop 1985;9(3):195–7.

20. Insall J, Salvati E. Patella position in the normal knee joint. Radiology 1971;101(1):101–4.

21. Koshino T, Sugimoto K. New measurement of patellar height in the knees of children using the epiphyseal line midpoint. J Pediatr Orthop 1989; 9(2):216–8.

22. Grelsamer RP, Meadows S. The modified Insall-Salvati ratio for assessment of patellar height. Clin Orthop Relat Res 1992;(282):170–6.

23. Parikh S, Noyes FR. Patellofemoral disorders: role of computed tomography and magnetic resonance imaging in defining abnormal rotational lower limb alignment. Sports Health 2011;3(2):158–69.

24. Song EK, Seon JK, Kim MC, et al. Radiologic measurement of tibial tuberosity-trochlear groove (TT-TG) distance by lower extremity rotational profile computed tomography in Koreans. Clin Orthop Surg 2016;8(1):45–8.

25. Dickens AJ, Morrell NT, Doering A, et al. Tibial tubercle-trochlear groove distance: defining normal in a pediatric population. J Bone Joint Surg Am 2014;96(4):318–24.

26. Tensho K, Akaoka Y, Shimodaira H, et al. What components comprise the measurement of the tibial tuberosity-trochlear groove distance in a patellar dislocation population? J Bone Joint Surg Am 2015;97(17):1441–8.

27. Tensho K, Shimodaira H, Akaoka Y, et al. Lateralization of the tibial tubercle in recurrent patellar dislocation: verification using multiple methods to evaluate the tibial tubercle. J Bone Joint Surg Am 2018;100(9):e58.

28. Loeb AE, Tanaka MJ. The medial patellofemoral complex. Curr Rev Musculoskelet Med 2018;11(2):201–8.

29. Amis AA, Firer P, Mountney J, et al. Anatomy and biomechanics of the medial patellofemoral ligament. Knee 2003;10(3):215–20.

30. Chotel F, Berard J, Raux S. Patellar instability in children and adolescents. Orthop Traumatol Surg Res 2014;100(1 Suppl):S125–37.

31. DeFroda SF, Gil JA, Boulos A, et al. Diagnosis and management of traumatic patellar instability in the pediatric patient. Orthopedics 2017;40(5):e749–57.

32. Clark D, Metcalfe A, Wogan C, et al. Adolescent patellar instability: current concepts review. Bone Joint J 2017;99-B(2):159–70.

33. Dejour DH. The patellofemoral joint and its historical roots: the Lyon School of Knee Surgery. Knee Surg Sports Traumatol Arthrosc 2013;21(7):1482–94.

34. Thompson P, Metcalfe AJ. Current concepts in the surgical management of patellar instability. Knee 2019;26(6):1171–81.

35. von Engelhardt LV, Raddatz M, Bouillon B, et al. How reliable is MRI in diagnosing cartilaginous lesions in patients with first and recurrent lateral patellar dislocations? BMC Musculoskelet Disord 2010;11:149.

36. Jain NP, Khan N, Fithian DC. A treatment algorithm for primary patellar dislocations. Sports Health 2011;3(2):170–4.

37. Ye Q, Yu T, Wu Y, et al. Patellar instability: the reliability of magnetic resonance imaging measurement parameters. BMC Musculoskelet Disord 2019;20(1):317.

38. Joseph S, Cheng C, Solomito M, et al. Lateral patellar inclination in children and adolescents: modified measurement technique to characterize patellar instability. Orthop J Sports Med 2019;7(3 suppl 1). 2325967119S2325900091.

39. Joseph S, Cheng C, Solomito M, et al. Lateral trochlear inclination angle in children and adolescents: modified measurement technique to characterize patellar instability. Orthop J Sports Med 2019;7(3 suppl 1). 2325967119S2325900146.

40. Yue RA, Arendt EA, Tompkins MA. Patellar height measurements on radiograph and magnetic resonance imaging in patellar instability and control patients. J knee Surg 2017;30(9):943–50.

41. Liu JN, Steinhaus ME, Kalbian IL, et al. Patellar instability management: a survey of the international patellofemoral study group. Am J Sports Med 2018;46(13):3299–306.

42. Minkowitz R, Inzerillo C, Sherman OH. Patella instability. Bull NYU Hosp Jt Dis 2007;65(4):280–93.

43. Pedowitz JM, Edmonds EW, Chambers HG, et al. Recurrence of patellar instability in adolescents undergoing surgery for osteochondral defects without concomitant ligament reconstruction. Am J Sports Med 2019;47(1):66–70.

44. Seeley MA, Knesek M, Vanderhave KL. Osteochondral injury after acute patellar dislocation in children and adolescents. J Pediatr Orthop 2013; 33(5):511–8.

45. Garth WP Jr, Pomphrey M Jr, Merrill K. Functional treatment of patellar dislocation in an athletic population. Am J Sports Med 1996;24(6):785–91.

46. Gigante A, Pasquinelli FM, Paladini P, et al. The effects of patellar taping on patellofemoral incongruence. A computed tomography study. Am J Sports Med 2001;29(1):88–92.

47. Schlichte LM, Sidharthan S, Green DW, et al. Pediatric management of recurrent patellar instability. Sports Med Arthrosc Rev 2019;27(4): 171–80.

48. Bremer Hinkel B, Arendt EA. Lateral retinaculum lengthening or release. Oper Tech Sports Med 2015;23(2):100–6.

49. Fithian DC, Paxton EW, Post WR, et al, International Patellofemoral Study Group. Lateral retinacular release: a survey of the International Patellofemoral Study Group. Arthroscopy 2004; 20(5):463–8.

50. Magnussen RA, De Simone V, Lustig S, et al. Treatment of patella alta in patients with episodic patellar dislocation: a systematic review. Knee Surg Sports Traumatol Arthrosc 2014;22(10):2545–50.

51. Payne J, Rimmke N, Schmitt LC, et al. The incidence of complications of tibial tubercle osteotomy: a systematic review. Arthroscopy 2015;31(9): 1819–25.

52. Andrish J. Surgical options for patellar stabilization in the skeletally immature patient. Sports Med Arthrosc Rev 2007;15(2):82–8.

53. Caton JH, Dejour D. Tibial tubercle osteotomy in patello-femoral instability and in patellar height abnormality. Int Orthop 2010;34(2):305–9.

54. Mayer C, Magnussen RA, Servien E, et al. Patellar tendon tenodesis in association with tibial tubercle distalization for the treatment of episodic patellar dislocation with patella alta. Am J Sports Med 2012;40(2):346–51.

55. Arendt EA, Fithian DC, Cohen E. Current concepts of lateral patella dislocation. Clin Sports Med 2002; 21(3):499–519.

56. Camp CL, Krych AJ, Dahm DL, et al. Medial patellofemoral ligament repair for recurrent patellar dislocation. Am J Sports Med 2010;38(11):2248–54.

57. Ostermeier S, Holst M, Bohnsack M, et al. Dynamic measurement of patellofemoral contact pressure following reconstruction of the medial patellofemoral ligament: an in vitro study. Clin Biomech (Bristol, Avon) 2007;22(3):327–35.

58. Bicos J, Carofino B, Andersen M, et al. Patellofemoral forces after medial patellofemoral ligament reconstruction: a biomechanical analysis. J knee Surg 2006;19(4):317–26.

59. McNeilan RJ, Everhart JS, Mescher PK, et al. Graft choice in isolated medial patellofemoral ligament reconstruction: a systematic review with meta-analysis of rates of recurrent instability and patient-reported outcomes for autograft, allograft, and synthetic options. Arthroscopy 2018;34(4): 1340–54.

60. Steiner TM, Torga-Spak R, Teitge RA. Medial patellofemoral ligament reconstruction in patients with lateral patellar instability and trochlear dysplasia. Am J Sports Med 2006;34(8):1254–61.

61. Nelitz M, Dreyhaupt J, Reichel H, et al. Anatomic reconstruction of the medial patellofemoral ligament in children and adolescents with open growth plates: surgical technique and clinical outcome. Am J Sports Med 2013;41(1):58–63.

62. Schottle PB, Schmeling A, Rosenstiel N, et al. Radiographic landmarks for femoral tunnel placement in medial patellofemoral ligament reconstruction. Am J Sports Med 2007;35(5):801–4.

63. Nelitz M, Dornacher D, Dreyhaupt J, et al. The relation of the distal femoral physis and the medial patellofemoral ligament. Knee Surg Sports Traumatol Arthrosc 2011;19(12):2067–71.

64. Gausden EB, Fabricant PD, Taylor SA, et al. Medial patellofemoral reconstruction in children and adolescents. JBJS Rev 2015;3(10). 01874474-201510000-00001.

65. Spang RC, Tepolt FA, Paschos NK, et al. Combined reconstruction of the medial patellofemoral ligament (MPFL) and medial quadriceps tendon-femoral ligament (MQTFL) for patellar instability in children and adolescents: surgical technique and outcomes. J Pediatr Orthop 2019;39(1):e54–61.

66. Joseph SM, Fulkerson JP. Medial quadriceps tendon femoral ligament reconstruction technique and surgical anatomy. Arthrosc Tech 2019;8(1): e57–64.

67. Hiemstra LA, Kerslake S, Loewen M, et al. Effect of trochlear dysplasia on outcomes after isolated soft tissue stabilization for patellar instability. Am J Sports Med 2016;44(6):1515–23.

68. Gravesen KS, Kallemose T, Blond L, et al. Persistent morbidity after Medial Patellofemoral Ligament Reconstruction - A registry study with an eight-year follow-up on a nationwide cohort from 1996 to 2014. Knee 2019;26(1):20–5.

69. Balcarek P, Rehn S, Howells NR, et al. Results of medial patellofemoral ligament reconstruction compared with trochleoplasty plus individual extensor apparatus balancing in patellar instability caused by severe trochlear dysplasia: a systematic review and meta-analysis. Knee Surg Sports Traumatol Arthrosc 2017;25(12):3869–77.

70. Fulkerson JP. Anteromedialization of the tibial tuberosity for patellofemoral malalignment. Clin Orthop Relat Res 1983;177:176–81.

71. Grimm NL, Lazarides AL, Amendola A. Tibial tubercle osteotomies: a review of a treatment for recurrent patellar instability. Curr Rev Musculoskelet Med 2018;11(2):266–71.

72. Damasena I, Blythe M, Wysocki D, et al. Medial patellofemoral ligament reconstruction combined with distal realignment for recurrent dislocations

of the patella: 5-year results of a randomized controlled trial. Am J Sports Med 2017;45(2): 369–76.

73. Luhmann SJ, O'Donnell JC, Fuhrhop S. Outcomes after patellar realignment surgery for recurrent patellar instability dislocations: a minimum 3-year follow-up study of children and adolescents. J Pediatr Orthop 2011;31(1):65–71.

74. Longo UG, Rizzello G, Ciuffreda M, et al. Elmslie-trillat, maquet, fulkerson, roux goldthwait, and other distal realignment procedures for the management of patellar dislocation: systematic review and quantitative synthesis of the literature. Arthroscopy 2016;32(5):929–43.

75. Sillanpaa P, Mattila VM, Visuri T, et al. Ligament reconstruction versus distal realignment for patellar dislocation. Clin Orthop Relat Res 2008;466(6):1475–84.

76. Post WR, Fithian DC. Patellofemoral Instability: A Consensus Statement From the AOSSM/PFF Patellofemoral Instability Workshop. Orthop J Sports Med 2018;6(1). 2325967117750352.

77. Balcarek P, Zimmermann F. Deepening trochleoplasty and medial patellofemoral ligament reconstruction normalize patellotrochlear congruence in severe trochlear dysplasia. Bone Joint J 2019;101-b(3):325–30.

78. Metcalfe AJ, Clark DA, Kemp MA, et al. Trochleoplasty with a flexible osteochondral flap: results from an 11-year series of 214 cases. Bone Joint J 2017;99-b(3):344–50.

79. Camathias C, Studer K, Kiapour A, et al. Trochleoplasty as a solitary treatment for recurrent patellar dislocation results in good clinical outcome in adolescents. Am J Sports Med 2016;44(11):2855–63.

80. McNamara I, Bua N, Smith TO, et al. Deepening trochleoplasty with a thick osteochondral flap for patellar instability: clinical and functional outcomes at a mean 6-year follow-up. Am J Sports Med 2015; 43(11):2706–13.

81. LaPrade RF, Cram TR, James EW, et al. Trochlear dysplasia and the role of trochleoplasty. Clin Sports Med 2014;33(3):531–45.

82. Dejour D, Byn P, Ntagiopoulos PG. The Lyon's sulcus-deepening trochleoplasty in previous unsuccessful patellofemoral surgery. Int Orthop 2013; 37(3):433–9.

83. Hiemstra LA, Peterson D, Youssef M, et al. Trochleoplasty provides good clinical outcomes and an acceptable complication profile in both short and long-term follow-up. Knee Surg Sports Traumatol Arthrosc 2018;27(9):2967–83.

84. Longo UG, Vincenzo C, Mannering N, et al. Trochleoplasty techniques provide good clinical results in patients with trochlear dysplasia. Knee Surg Sports Traumatol Arthrosc 2017;26(9):2640–58.

85. Nelitz M, Williams SR. [Combined trochleoplasty and medial patellofemoral ligament reconstruction for patellofemoral instability]. Oper Orthop Traumatol 2015;27(6):495–504.

86. Banke IJ, Kohn LM, Meidinger G, et al. Combined trochleoplasty and MPFL reconstruction for treatment of chronic patellofemoral instability: a prospective minimum 2-year follow-up study. Knee Surg Sports Traumatol Arthrosc 2014; 22(11):2591–8.

87. Ntagiopoulos PG, Byn P, Dejour D. Midterm results of comprehensive surgical reconstruction including sulcus-deepening trochleoplasty in recurrent patellar dislocations with high-grade trochlear dysplasia. Am J Sports Med 2013;41(5):998–1004.

88. Nelitz M, Dreyhaupt J, Lippacher S. Combined trochleoplasty and medial patellofemoral ligament reconstruction for recurrent patellar dislocations in severe trochlear dysplasia: a minimum 2-year follow-up study. Am J Sports Med 2013;41(5): 1005–12.

89. Testa EA, Camathias C, Amsler F, et al. Surgical treatment of patellofemoral instability using trochleoplasty or MPFL reconstruction: a systematic review. Knee Surg Sports Traumatol Arthrosc 2017; 25(8):2309–20.

90. Song GY, Hong L, Zhang H, et al. Trochleoplasty versus nontrochleoplasty procedures in treating patellar instability caused by severe trochlear dysplasia. Arthroscopy 2014;30(4):523–32.

91. Nelitz M, Dreyhaupt J, Williams SRM. No growth disturbance after trochleoplasty for recurrent patellar dislocation in adolescents with open growth plates. Am J Sports Med 2018;46(13):3209–16.

92. Holliday CL, Hiemstra LA, Kerslake S, et al. Relationship between anatomical risk factors, articular cartilage lesions, and patient outcomes following medial patellofemoral ligament reconstruction. Cartilage 2019. https://doi.org/10.1177/1947603519894728. 1947603519894728.

93. Mofidi A, Veravalli K, Jinnah RH, et al. Association and impact of patellofemoral dysplasia on patellofemoral arthropathy and arthroplasty. Knee 2014; 21(2):509–13.

94. Jungmann PM, Tham SC, Liebl H, et al. Association of trochlear dysplasia with degenerative abnormalities in the knee: data from the Osteoarthritis Initiative. Skeletal Radiol 2013;42(10):1383–92.

95. Ali SA, Helmer R, Terk MR. Analysis of the patellofemoral region on MRI: association of abnormal trochlear morphology with severe cartilage defects. AJR Am J Roentgenol 2010;194(3):721–7.

96. Schottle PB, Schell H, Duda G, et al. Cartilage viability after trochleoplasty. Knee Surg Sports Traumatol Arthrosc 2007;15(2):161–7.

97. Amis AA, Oguz C, Bull AM, et al. The effect of trochleoplasty on patellar stability and kinematics: a biomechanical study in vitro. J Bone Joint Surg Br 2008;90(7):864–9.

Gymnast's Wrist (Distal Radial Physeal Stress Syndrome)

Benjamin Mauck, MD*, Derek Kelly, MD,
Benjamin Sheffer, MD, Anna Rambo, MD,
James H. Calandruccio, MD

KEYWORDS

• Distal radial physis • Overuse injuries • Physeal closure • Gymnast's wrist • Stress syndrome

KEY POINTS

- The distal radial physis is a common site for injury in gymnasts because of the significant amount of load applied during upper extremity weight-bearing. Wrist pain has been reported in up to 88% of gymnasts.
- The wrist is subjected to forces in gymnastics that can exceed twice the body weight, and rates of loading up to 16 times body weight have been reported. In addition to high-impact loading, the wrist is exposed to repetitive motion, axial compression, torsional forces, and distraction.
- Radiographic criteria for the diagnosis of stress injuries to the distal radial physis include widening of the physis, especially volarly and radially; cystic changes of the metaphyseal aspect of the physis; a beaked distal volar and radial physis; and haziness within the physis.
- Initial treatment for most patients is rest from the offending activity until the wrist is pain-free, followed by a gradual return to activity; operative intervention generally is indicated for more severe growth arrest.

In 2017, there were nearly 5 million participants in gymnastics aged 6 years and older[1]; elite gymnasts, however, may begin training as early as 4 or 5 years of age. An awareness of overuse injuries among young athletes is increasing. Early sport specialization and increasing training hours have contributed to higher rates of overuse injuries in young athletes. In numerous youth sports, for example, gymnastics and rowing, overuse wrist injuries are a well-known problem, with prevalence rates for wrist pain of 32% to 73%.[2–4]

The distal radial physis is a common site for injury in gymnasts because of the significant amount of load applied during upper extremity weight-bearing. There have been multiple series reporting stress injuries to the distal radial physes.[5–11] The cause likely is repeated injury to the physis from compression, distraction, and torsion forces.[11] The cause of physeal injury also may be from compromise of the blood supply to the metaphysis and/or epiphysis,[12] which can lead to abnormal endochondral ossification.

Unlike most other sports, in gymnastics the upper extremities are used for weight-bearing. The wrist is subjected to forces in gymnastics that can exceed twice the body weight, and rates of loading up to 16 times body weight have been reported.[3,11,13] Given these high-impact loads, the wrist is the most frequently injured site in the upper extremity of female gymnasts.[3,11,13] In addition to high-impact loading, the wrist is exposed to repetitive motion, axial compression, torsional forces, and distraction.[11,14,15] Combining these forces with varying degrees of ulnar and radial deviation and hyperextension predisposes the wrist to higher rates of injury during gymnastics. DiFiori and colleagues[8] estimated that 46% to 79% of

Department of Orthopaedic Surgery and Biomechanical Engineering, University of Tennessee-Campbell Clinic, Memphis, TN, USA
* Corresponding author. 1458 West Poplar Avenue, Suite 100, Collierville, TN 38017.
E-mail address: bmauck@campbellclinic.com

Orthop Clin N Am 51 (2020) 493–497
https://doi.org/10.1016/j.ocl.2020.06.012
0030-5898/20/© 2020 Elsevier Inc. All rights reserved.

gymnasts experience wrist pain, whereas according to Dobyns and Gables,[16] up to 88% of gymnasts experience wrist pain. In a study by DiFiori and colleagues,[17] 83% of gymnasts between 10 and 14 years of age had wrist pain, compared with 44% for those outside of that age range. Fifty-one percent (30 of 59) had findings of stress injury to the distal radial physis of at least a grade 2; 7% (4) had frank widening of the growth plate.

Cross-sectional surveys indicate that approximately 45% of gymnasts report pain of at least 6 months' duration.[14,17] In a prospective cohort study of young, competitive gymnasts observed for 1 year, 89% of those with wrist pain at the beginning of the study had symptoms 1 year later.[17]

CLINICAL PRESENTATION

Skeletally immature gymnasts with chronic wrist pain typically describe a dorsally located, aching pain that is provoked with gymnastics activities. The typical patient with a distal radial stress fracture is a 12- to 14-year-old girl who is participating in gymnastics more than 35 hours each week. Symptoms begin at the onset of the offending activity and worsen during the activity. On examination, tenderness to direct pressure at the wrist over the distal radius physis may be detected. The pain also can sometimes be reproduced with hyperextension of the wrist or asking the athlete to perform push-ups or handstands while in the office. Gymnast's wrist can be confused with tendonitis of the extensor tendons of the wrist; however, usually with tendonitis, the athlete will have pain with direct palpation of the tendons, as well as resisted extension of the wrist without pressure to the distal radius. Other causes also may be mistaken for gymnast's wrist (Box 1).

Factors predisposing gymnasts to wrist pain include improper equipment, incorrect techniques, previous injury, delayed skeletal maturity, and growth spurts because of the transient weakness in the physis.[18] Peak growth velocity occurs in men and women at approximately 13.5 years and 11.5 years, respectively.

Rettig divided distal radial physeal injury into 3 stages. In stage 1, the diagnosis is made clinically before radiographic abnormalities.[10] Gradual return to participation can begin once symptoms cease. Stage 2 demonstrates radiographic radial physeal changes as described previously. Return to competition is much longer and can be up to 2 to 4 months. Stage 3 has the same clinical features as stage 2 with ulnar positive variance on radiographs.

Often the pain will go unreported for weeks to months, because of the athlete's desire to continue participating. The subjectivity of pain perception may be an obstacle when it comes to a pediatric athletic population. Nemeth and colleagues[19] observed in a group of 68 Olympic level patients aged 6 to 13 years that the older ones (older than 11 years) had a better characterization of pain and understanding of its implications than the younger ones, mostly 6 to 8 years old, many of whom understand pain as something to be overcome to improve performance, as if it were part of the training. Young gymnasts often do not even report painful incidents of the wrist to their coaches even if they occur frequently.[20] Studies of young athletes have shown that many view competing or training while in pain as normal.[21,22] Kox and colleagues[22] found that limitations in daily life activities can prompt young athletes to seek medical care more often than pain during training or competition and may, therefore, indicate overuse wrist injury in this population. They advised physicians and trainers to inquire specifically about limitations and pain during daily life activities.

RADIOGRAPHIC EVALUATION

Radiographic criteria for the diagnosis of stress injuries to the distal radial physis include widening of the physis, especially volarly and radially; cystic changes of the metaphyseal aspect of the physis; a beaked distal volar and radial physis; and haziness within the physis[23] (Fig. 1).

Newer techniques such as fat-suppressed 3-dimensional spoiled gradient-recalled echo imaging can identify premature physeal bony bridge formation and provide information on the exact location and size of a bony bridge, which can be used for surgical planning.[24,25] A large and central bridge leads to length discrepancy, whereas a small and peripheral bridge causes an angular deformity.[24] If less than 50% of the physis is

Box 1
Other causes of wrist pain in young athletes
Tendonitis
Scaphoid fracture
Scaphoid/ulnar impaction syndrome
Physeal or metaphyseal traumatic fracture
Congenital deformity (eg, Madelung deformity, radioulnar synostosis)
TFCC tears
Osteonecrosis of capitate
Ganglia

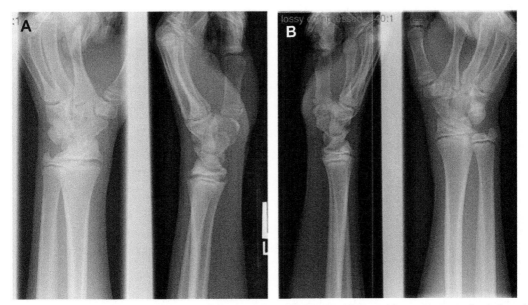

Fig. 1. (A) Lateral and oblique radiographs of distal radial stress injury in a 13-year-old gymnast; note distal physeal widening most pronounced volarly and radially. (B) Comparison radiograph of the asymptomatic wrist with normal-appearing distal radial morphology. (From Webb BG, Rettig LA. Gymnastic wrist injuries. Curr Sports Med Rep 2008; 7:289-295.)

involved, the growth arrest can be treated with bridge excision and interposition.

ULNAR VARIANCE

Ulnar variance refers to the relative length of the ulna with respect to the radius, determined at the carpal surface. Neutral variance occurs when the bones are of equal length. It is defined as negative variance when the ulna is shorter than the radius and positive variance when the ulna is longer than the radius (Fig. 2). Ulnar variance affects the distribution of force across the wrist, and a significant amount of research has been conducted to investigate the relationship between ulnar variance and distal radial stress injuries.[13,26–28] Experimental studies suggest that the load is increased across the radius as the ulnar variance becomes more negative.[12] As a general rule, the ulnar variance in children with open physes is usually negative. Therefore, it can be inferred that it is likely that the loading across the radius is significant in young, skeletally immature gymnasts who already have negative ulnar variances. There are reports showing greater prevalence of relative and absolute positive ulnar variance in gymnasts compared with nongymnasts in both skeletally mature and immature gymnasts.[26–28] Over time, 2 conflicting longitudinal studies of ulnar variance in young gymnasts show different trends in ulnar variance. One suggests increasing negative ulnar variance,[29] and the other suggests significantly more positive variance over time.[27]

In a sample of young gymnasts (mean age, 9.3 years), the mean ulnar variance was significantly greater than in nongymnasts, although all gymnasts had an ulnar variance that was within the range of normal for their age.[17] In

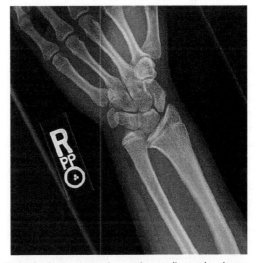

Fig. 2. Anteroposterior wrist radiograph demonstrating positive ulnar variance in a young gymnast. (From Benjamin HJ, Engel SC, Chudzik D. Wrist pain in gymnasts: a review of common overuse wrist pathology in the gymnastics athlete. Curr Sports Med Rep 2017; 16:322-329.)

fact, data show that the mean ulnar variance among gymnasts is in the upper range of normal. However, some measurements may be clearly beyond the normal range. In a study of elite gymnasts, 19.8% of skeletally mature subjects and 11.5% of skeletally immature subjects had ulnar variance measurements in excess of the upper limits of the 95% confidence intervals for a reference sample.[30] Such findings would raise clinical concern, especially in those with symptoms of wrist pain.

Ulnar overgrowth has been associated with ulnocarpal impaction syndrome, abnormal wrist function, distal radioulnar joint instability, and significant impairment of activities of daily living (DiFiori). A Madelung-like deformity, where the articular surface of the distal radius is directed volar and ulnar, has been described with premature closure of the ulnar aspect of the distal radius physis.[11,28,29]

Altered length or angular relationship between the radius and ulna also may lead to decreased range of motion and strength.[25] The most common indication for surgery is symptomatic abnormal ulnar variance or asymptomatic abnormal variance with substantial growth remaining. Rather than increasing the overall length of the extremity, the primary goal of surgery is to create a level joint.

TREATMENT

Treatment varies by site and type of arrest. Initial treatment of most patients is rest from the offending activity until the wrist is pain-free, followed by a gradual return to activity. DiFiori recommended refraining from compression loading of the wrist for 6 weeks.[28] If at that time the physical examination is unremarkable and imaging studies show resolution of the physeal injury, training can resume. Although biomechanical[31] and clinical[32] study has indicated that bracing may provide some protection from acute injuries, its effectiveness in repetitive loading of the wrist has not been reported.

Operative intervention generally is indicated for more severe growth arrest; techniques include epiphysiodesis, lengthening osteotomy, shortening osteotomy, excision of physeal bar or bone fragment, angular correction osteotomy, and rarely creation of single bone forearm for a significant deformity (Box 2). With a partial physeal arrest, if a distinct bar can be identified and is less than 50% of the physeal surface, bar excision is recommended. If the partial physeal arrest is indistinct or involves more than 50% of the physeal surface, completion of the arrest with an

---

Box 2
Surgical treatment of distal radial physeal arrest

- Excision of physeal bar
- Distal ulnar epiphysiodesis
- Ulnar lengthening osteotomy with or without autograft
- Ulnar shortening osteotomy with or without distal ulnar epiphysiodesis
- Distal radial epiphysiodesis
- Radial lengthening osteotomy, distal ulnar epiphysiodesis
- Distal radius volar fragment excision with radiocarpal reduction/pinning
- Radial lengthening osteotomy, distal ulnar epiphysiodesis,
- Radial lengthening osteotomy, distal ulnar epiphysiodesis, distal radial epiphysiodesis
- Radial shortening osteotomy and ulnar lengthening osteotomy
- Wrist arthroscopy, ulnar shortening osteotomy
- Wrist arthroscopy, ulnar shortening osteotomy, distal ulnar epiphysiodesis

Adapted from Gauger EM, Casnovsky LL, Gauger EJ, et al: Acquired upper extremity growth arrest. Orthopedics 2017; 40:e95-e103.

---

epiphysiodesis is recommended. For the distal radius and ulna, treatment should be focused on achieving joint leveling (neutral ulnar variance). Before skeletal maturity, epiphysiodesis of the longer bone is recommended for children older than 12 years and stapling of the physis of the longer bone for children younger than 12 years. After skeletal maturity, this can be achieved by lengthening the radius or by shortening the ulna.

SUMMARY

The long-term consequences of overuse wrist injuries, such as distal radial physeal arrest, include degenerative conditions that often cause pain and functional limitations. In the more immediate stage of many overuse injuries, early diagnosis can promote quicker care and recovery and thus faster return to play. Less time lost to injury can be very important in maintaining an athlete's quality of life.

DISCLOSURE

Drs. Mauck, Kelly, Sheffer, and Calandruccio disclose publishing royalties from Elsevier; Dr. Mauck discloses consultant fees from Olympus Endoscopy. No other conflicts exist.

REFERENCES

1. Statisa.com. Available at: https://www.statista.com/statistics/191908/participants-in-gymnastics-in-the-us. Accessed May 31, 2020.
2. Caine D, Roy S, Singer K, et al. Stress changes of the distal radial growth plate: a radiographic survey of 60 young competitive gymnasts and an epidemiologic review of the related literature. Am J Sports Med 1992;20:290–8.
3. Gauger EM, Casnovsky LL, Gauger EJ, et al. Acquired upper extremity growth arrest. Orthopedics 2017;40:e95–103.
4. Jayanthi NA, LaBella CR, Fischer D, et al. Sports-specialized intensive training and the risk of injury in young athletes: a clinical case control study. Am J Sports Med 2015;43(4):794–801.
5. Albanese SA, Palmer AK, Kerr DR, et al. Wrist pain and distal growth plat3e closure in gymnasts. J Pediatr Orthop 1989;9:23–8.
6. Caine D, Knutzen K, Howe W, et al. A three-year epidemiological study of injuries affecting young female gymnasts. Phys Ther Sport 2003;4:10–23.
7. Chawla A, Wiesler ER. Nonspecific wrist pain in gymnasts and cheerleaders. Clin Sports Med 2015;34:143–9.
8. DiFiori JP, Caine DJ, Malina RM. Wrist pain, distal radial physeal injury, and ulnar variance the young gymnast. Am J Sports Med 2006;34:840–9.
9. Guerra MRV, Estelles JRD, Abdouni YA, et al. Frequency of wrist growth plate injury in young gymnasts at a training center. Acta Orthop Bras 2016;24:204–7.
10. Rettig AC. Athletic injuries of the wrist and hand: part II: overuse injuries of the wrist and traumatic injuries of the hand. Am J Sports Med 2004;32:262–73.
11. Abzug JM, Little K, Kozin SH. Physeal arrest of the distal radius. J Am Acad Orthop Surg 2014;22:381–9.
12. Jaramillo D, Laor T, Zaleske DJ. Indirect trauma to the growth plate: results of MR imaging after epiphyseal and metaphyseal injury in rabbits. Radiology 1993;187:171–8.
13. Benjamin HJ, Engel SC, Chudzik D. Wrist pain in gymnasts: a review of common overuse pathology in the gymnastics athlete. Curr Sports Med Rep 2017;16:322–9.
14. DiFiori JP, Puffer JC, Mandelbaum BR, et al. Factors associated with wrist pain in the young gymnast. Am J Sports Med 1996;24:9–14.
15. Kox LS, Kuijer PPFM, Kerkhoffs GMMJ, et al. Prevalence, incidence and risk factors for overuse injuries of the wrist in young athletes: a systematic review. Br J Sports Med 2015;49(18):1189–96.
16. Dobyns JH, Gabel GT. Gymnast's wrist. Hand Clin 1990;6:493–505.
17. DiFiori JP, Puffer JC, Aish B, et al. Wrist pain, distal radial physeal injury, and ulnar variance in young gymnasts: does a relationship exist? Am J Sports Med 2002;30:879–85.
18. Hart E, Meehan WP 3rd, Bae DS, et al. The young injured gymnast: a literature review and discission. Curr Sports Med Rep 2018;17:366–75.
19. Nemeth R, Von Baeyer C, Rocha EM. Young gymnasts' understanding of sport-related pain: a contribution to prevention of injury. Child Care Health Dev 2005;31:615–25.
20. Valovich Mc Leod TC, Bay RC, Parsons JT, et al. Recent injury and health-related quality of life in adolescent athletes. J Athl Train 2009;44:603.
21. Coates C, McMurth CM, Lingley-Pottie P, et al. The prevalence of painful incidents among young recreational gymnasts. Pain Res Manag 2010;15:179–84.
22. Kox KS, Opperman J, Kuijer PPFM, et al. A hidden mismatch between experiences of young athletes with overuse injuries of the wrist and sports physicians' perceptions: a focus group study. BMC Musculoskelet Disord 2019;20:235–45.
23. Webb BG, Rettig LA. Gymnastic wrist injuries. Curr Sports Med Rep 2008;7:289–95.
24. Ecklund K, Jaramillo D. Patterns of premature physeal arrest: MR imaging of 111 children. AJR Am J Roentgenol 2002;178:967–72.
25. Kraan RBJ, Kox LS, Mens MA, et al. Damage of the distal radial physis in young gymnassts: can three-dimensional assessment of physeal volume of MRI serve as a biomarker? Eur Radiol 2019;29:6364–71.
26. DiFiori JP, Puffer JC, Mandelbaum BR, et al. Distal radial growth plate injury and positive ulnar variance. Am J Sports Med 1997;25:763–8.
27. DiFiori JP, Puffer JC, Dorey F. Ulnar variance in young gymnasts: a three-year study. Med Sci Sports Exerc 2001;33:S223.
28. DiFiori JP. Overuse injury and the young athlete: the case of chronic wrist pain in gymnasts. Curr Sports Med Rep 2006;5:165.
29. Claessens AL, Lefevre J, Beunen G, et al. Physique as a risk factor for ulnar variance in elite female gymnasts. Med Sci Sports Exerc 1996;28:560–9.
30. Claessens AL, Lefevre J, Philippaerts R, et al. The ulnar variance phenomenon: a study in young gymnasts. In: Armstrong N, Kirby B, Welsman J, editors. Children and exercise XIX. London: E & FN Spon; 1997. p. 537–41.
31. Grant-Ford M, Sitler MR, Kozin SH, et al. Effect of a prophylactic brace on wrist and ulnocarpal joint biomechanics in a cadaveric model. Am J Sports Med 2003;31:736.
32. Trevithick B, Mellifont R, Sayers M. Wrist pain in gymnasts: efficacy of a wrist brace to decrease wrist pain while performing gymnastics. J Hand Ther 2019;4:S0894-1130(18):30291–6.

Hand and Wrist

An Evidence-Based Review of Overuse Wrist Injuries in Athletes

Sierra G. Phillips, MD[1]

KEYWORDS
• Overuse injuries • Wrist injuries • Athletes • Tendinopathy • Impaction syndromes • Wrist impingement

KEY POINTS
• Overuse injuries are a common source of wrist pain in athletes of all competitive levels.
• Overuse wrist injuries may result in tendinopathies or osteoarticular issues, such as impaction syndromes, impingement syndromes, and physeal stress injuries.
• Most of these conditions can be treated successfully with conservative measures, such as activity modification, immobilization or bracing, anti-inflammatory medications, therapy, and corticosteroid injections.
• Published evidence supports favorable outcomes after treatment of overuse injuries, even if surgical intervention is required.

INTRODUCTION

Injuries to the wrist and hand commonly occur in professional, amateur, and recreational athletes. They comprise approximately 25% of all sports-related injuries and can be linked to sports-specific activities.[1–4] Many of these injuries are due to overuse from repetitive motions as opposed to an acute traumatic event. Overuse injuries are caused by recurrent microtrauma that overwhelms local tissues' ability to fully heal and often can be seen in both contact sports and noncontact sports. When treating an athlete with an overuse injury of the wrist, there are various structures that can be pathologic, including bones, joints, tendons, ligaments, soft tissue, or any combination.[5]

Fortunately, athletes with overuse injuries of the wrist only occasionally have to refrain from participating in their sport because they can be treated with a spectrum of conservative measures. Of special note in this patient population is the use of corticosteroid injections (CSIs) and the implications this may have if highly competitive athletes are being tested for performance-enhancing drugs. Due to the localized nature of CSI for wrist pathology, it is unlikely that any effects from an overall performance standpoint would occur. It is important, however, for athletes to be aware of the testing parameters to which they are subject. If conservative treatment, including CSIs, fails, there often are curative minor surgical procedures that can be done under local anesthesia, with or without sedation.

TENDINOPATHIES
de Quervain Tenosynovitis

The most diagnosed tendinopathy of the wrist involves the first dorsal extensor compartment, which includes the abductor pollicis longus (APL) and the extensor pollicis brevis (EPB) tendons. This entity is referred to as de Quervain tenosynovitis, and it is a common source of radial-sided wrist pain in athletes. It affects, in particular, those participating in sports who require forceful grasping while in ulnar deviation, such as tennis, golf, or rowing. Development of de Quervain tenosynovitis has been

Department of Orthopaedic Surgery and Biomedical Engineering, University of Tennessee-Campbell Clinic, 1211 Union Avenue, Suite 510, Memphis TN 38104, USA
[1]Present Address: 1400 S Germantown Rd, Germantown, TN 38138.
E-mail address: Sierragphillips@gmail.com

Orthop Clin N Am 51 (2020) 499–509
https://doi.org/10.1016/j.ocl.2020.06.007

linked to poor technique and mechanics.[6–8] Additionally, volleyball players with increased training times also are at risk due to repetitive impact of the ball on the radial wrist.[9] The pathology arises from shearing forces and repetitive gliding of the APL and EBP tendons as they run through a fibro-osseous tunnel and over the radial styloid, which results in a myxoid degeneration of the tissues rather than acute inflammation.[10] The diagnosis is a clinical one. Patients typically present with a triad of swelling at the radial styloid, tenderness to palpation over the first dorsal compartment proximal to the tip of the styloid, and a positive Eichhoff and/or Finkelstein maneuver.[11] For the Eichhoff maneuver, patients are asked to grasp their flexed thumb into a clenched fist and an ulnar deviation force is applied to the wrist. For the Finkelstein maneuver, the thumb is passively flexed by the examiner and the wrist is ulnarly deviated.[12] Reproducible pain along the first dorsal compartment is considered a positive provocative maneuver for both. In 2014, a novel diagnostic examination maneuver called the wrist hyperflexion abduction of the thumb (WHAT) test was described and reported to have better sensitivity and specificity than the Eichhoff maneuver. With the wrist fully flexed, the examiner resists thumb abduction to reproduce pain along the APL and EPB tendons[13] (Fig. 1). Imaging is not used routinely for diagnosis. In a systematic review, McBain and colleagues[14] were unable to determine the accuracy of various imaging modalities (radiographs, ultrasound, magnetic resonance imaging [MRI], and scintigraphy) in de Quervain tenosynovitis due to a lack of sufficient published data; however, they did note that ultrasound was the imaging modality used most often. Ultrasound and MRI often can detect tenosynovial effusion, thickening of the retinaculum, and anatomic variants that can lead to refractory cases. Conservative treatment begins with cessation of the inciting activity, thumb spica splinting, and nonsteroidal anti-inflammatory medications. Meta-analyses have reported that CSIs are the most effective conservative treatment.[15,16] Oh and colleagues[17] demonstrated that CSIs are curative 73% of the time with 2 injections. A recent study compared the efficacy of CSIs with and without immobilization and noted that immobilization increases costs, can hinder activities of daily living and did not contribute to better outcomes.[18] Surgical release of the fibro-osseous roof of the first dorsal compartment, either open or endoscopically, can be curative in cases of failed

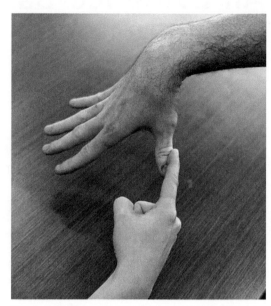

Fig. 1. WHAT examination maneuver for de Quervain tenosynovitis.

conservative measures, but a course of nonoperative treatment should be attempted first.[19] Care must be taken to protect the superficial radial nerve and to decompress any separate compartments and additional slips of tendon. Patients, especially athletes, must be counseled on postoperative expectations and rare but possible complications, including prolonged recovery with time out of sports, incomplete relief, transient superficial radial nerve irritation, and subluxation of the APL and EPB tendons. Generally, there is a period of 2 weeks to 3 weeks postoperatively before patients can return to normal activities, pending their comfort level.[20] A randomized controlled trial comparing endoscopic release of the first dorsal compartment (n = 27) to open release (n = 25), demonstrated that at 12 weeks after surgery the patients with endoscopic release had significantly better functional and pain scores. There was no difference in return-to-work times, and by week 24 the pain and functional scores had equalized and were significantly better than preoperative scores.[21]

Intersection Syndrome

Intersection syndrome, also called oarsman's wrist or squeaker's wrist, is a relatively uncommon overuse syndrome caused by repetitive wrist extension and radial deviation. It can be seen in athletes who participate in rowing, weightlifting, racquet sports, horseback riding, skiing, and cycling. Friction occurs as the first dorsal compartment tendons (APL and EPB) cross over the tendons of the second dorsal compartment, which include the extensor carpi radialis longus and extensor carpi radial brevis (ECRB).[2,8] Additionally, there may be a stenosing tenosynovitis within the second compartment itself.[22] Patients experience dorsoradial wrist pain with swelling, tenderness, and occasional crepitance on palpation approximately 4 cm to 6 cm proximal to Lister tubercle. Intersection syndrome also is more likely to occur in the dominant wrist.[23] It is important to differentiate intersection syndrome from de Quervain tenosynovitis on examination. Similarly, a clinical diagnosis of intersection syndrome usually is sufficient, negating the need for imaging studies in most cases.[6] If imaging is used for more complex presentations, ultrasound should be considered first line for its ability to complete a dynamic evaluation. Using ultrasound, Draghi and Bortolotto[24] were able to identify pathologic anatomy, including sheath variants and thickening. Additionally, a second location of distal intersection syndrome was described, where the second compartment runs under the third compartment consisting of the extensor pollicis longus.[24] MRI can identify peritendinous or subcutaneous edema, synovial effusions, and tendinosis.[25] Most symptoms resolve with activity modifications, immobilization of the wrist at neutral to 20° of extension, therapy, and anti-inflammatory medications. If needed, a CSI into the area of maximal tenderness can be helpful.[26] Although rare, if symptoms persist, a surgical release of the second extensor compartment with débridement of inflammatory tenosynovium can be completed, usually during the off-season. Postoperatively, patients need a brief period of immobilization followed by therapy, with the expectation of return to sports at 4 weeks to 6 weeks.[20] Although the rarity of surgery leads to a scarcity of literature, Hoy and colleagues[27] recently described aggressive surgical treatment of intersection syndrome in elite rowers to prevent time away from their sport. They noted that 5 of 6 elite rowers who had early surgical decompression returned to rowing at a median of 7 days postoperatively.

Extensor Carpi Ulnaris Tendinopathy

Conditions involving the extensor carpi ulnaris (ECU) tendon are the second most common wrist tendinopathy, causing ulnar-sided wrist pain in athletes who participate in rowing, golf, baseball, hockey, and racket sports.[2,28] It often is diagnosed in the nondominant hand of tennis players and is thought to be caused by the ulnar

deviation during a 2-handed backhand swing.[29] Any athlete who performs repetitive pronosupination with radial and ulnar deviation, however, is at risk. Numerous pathologies can affect the ECU tendon, including stenosing tenosynovitis, tendinosis and fraying, bony erosion of the sixth compartment floor, tendon subluxation, and rupture.[30,31] Subluxation and/or rupture can result from either an acute traumatic event or repetitive microtrauma. ECU tendinopathy manifests with vague dorsoulnar wrist swelling, tenderness along the course of the ECU tendon, and pain with resisted wrist extension and ulnar deviation. The ECU synergy maneuver can be used to help differentiate intra-articular pain from extra-articular pain by avoiding load to the ulnocarpal joint and triangular fibrocartilage complex (TFCC). This maneuver exploits an isometric contraction of the ECU and is performed with the elbow flexed at 90° and the forearm in full supination. The patient radially abducts the thumb against resistance with the examiner's finger on the patient's long finger for counterpressure (Fig. 2). Reproducible ulnar-sided wrist pain is considered a positive examination.[32] The sensitivity (73.7%) and specificity (85.7%) support this as a useful provocative maneuver.[33] To evaluate for ECU instability, also called snapping ECU, the patient is asked to flex and ulnarly deviate the wrist while in full supination. The acute angle made by the ECU should result in subluxation or dislocation if instability is present. The patient should also be evaluated for a TFCC injury because a peripheral tear can result in ECU irritation and symptomatology.[4] Routine use of imaging is not indicated, but ultrasound can demonstrate inflammatory changes and dynamic subluxation. Also, MRI can help identify subsheath injuries, tears in the ECU, and the anatomy of the ECU groove and rule out other structural abnormalities.[33] Initial treatment of stenosing tenosynovitis and tendinosis is conservative, with activity modification, anti-inflammatory medications, immobilization of the wrist, and therapy. Some practitioners prefer to immobilize with an above-elbow orthosis or cast to place the forearm in pronation, but there is no literature demonstrating a difference compared with wrist-only immobilization.[34,35] Treatment in a wrist orthosis can allow athletes to continue playing their sport.[6] CSI is another option, but care must be taken to avoid intratendinous injection that may lead to weakening of the tendon. Image guidance can help to confirm the appropriate injection site. For refractory cases, débridement of tenosynovitis or intrasubstance tendinosis, with or without surgical

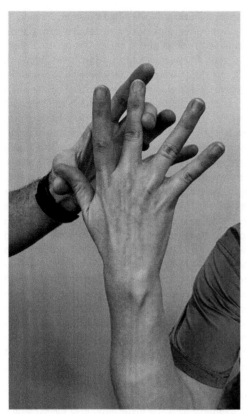

Fig. 2. ECU synergy examination maneuver for ECU tendinitis.

decompression, can be scheduled during the off-season. Decompression involves release of the sixth compartment through the radial aspect and into the fifth compartment, followed by extensor retinacular repair. If anomalous slips or extraneous septa between the ECU and the fifth compartment are encountered, they should be excised.[28]

For instability, the treatment is similar, but above-elbow immobilization is recommended to place the forearm in pronation, with the wrist extended and radially deviated using a Muenster-type orthosis.[36] There are reports of successful nonoperative treatments in elite tennis players who underwent 2 months to 3 months of immobilization, with return to play at 5 months to 6 months symptom-free.[29] With chronic instability, repair or reconstruction of the ECU subsheath is required. Repair can be accomplished through direct suture repair or approximation of the sheath to bone through bone tunnels. Reconstruction is achieved by using a strip of extensor retinaculum and can be done with or without groove deepening. In a cadaver model, groove deepening did not improve ECU stability compared with subsheath reconstruction.[37]

Postoperatively, patients should remain in a long arm splint for 2 weeks to 6 weeks, followed by therapy.[20,38] Projected return to play for elite athletes is 3 months with an accelerated program. Graham noted that in his experience, 25% of athletes return at 10 weeks to 12 weeks, 50% at 12 weeks to 14 weeks, and the remaining 25% after week 14.[38]

Flexor Carpi Ulnaris Tendinopathy

Overuse syndromes of the flexor carpi ulnaris (FCU) are fairly rare but can affect athletes participating in golf and racket sports.[5] The FCU tendon does not run in a sheath and, therefore, cannot develop stenosing tenosynovitis. Instead, FCU pathology can present as calcific tendonitis or noncalcific tendinopathy.[39] Athletes describe activity-related pain localized to the volar aspect of the ulnar wrist. Patients typically have tenderness 3 cm proximal to the insertion on the pisiform extending along the FCU tendon, and it is important to avoid compression of the pisotriquetral joint, which can be a different source of ulnar-sided wrist pain.[40] With calcific tendonitis, patients may have a moderate to severe inflammatory reaction with swelling and erythema similar to a gouty or infectious process. Imaging should include radiographs of the wrist to rule out calcific deposits within the FCU tendon and pisotriquetral arthritis. Ultrasonography and MRI can show peritendinous inflammatory changes, tendinosis, and calcific deposits.[41] Conservative treatment consists of splinting the wrist, anti-inflammatory medications, therapy, and CSIs. If symptoms do not resolve, surgical treatment involves débridement of the FCU tendon. Budoff and colleagues reported 5 patients with noncalcific FCU tendinopathy treated with intratendinous débridement of degenerative tissue through a longitudinal incision, followed by a side-to-side closure. Patients were splinted for 1 week and then allowed to progressively return to daily activities without therapy. All patients had complete or near-complete resolution of symptoms at 1-year follow-up. Additionally, the débrided tissue was noted to be angiofibroblastic hyperplasia, not acute inflammation, which could have implications in treatment strategies.[40] It may be more beneficial to treat noncalcific tendinopathy similar to lateral epicondylitis and focus more on stretching and strengthening than on anti-inflammatory modalities.[20]

Flexor Carpi Radialis Tendinopathy

The flexor carpi radialis (FCR) tendon is infrequently affected by tendinopathy, but its anatomy can predispose it to problems. Distally, it passes over the distal pole of the scaphoid, making an acute angle to enter a tight fibro-osseous tunnel bordered mostly by the trapezium, where the tendon occupies 90% of the space.[42,43] Acute overstretching or chronic wrist flexion leads to tendinopathic symptoms and is seen mostly in volleyball, basketball, water polo, golf, stick sports, and racquet sports.[4,20] FCR tendinopathy also is associated with peritrapezial arthritis because of its proximity, but this is less likely to be the offending agent in younger athletes.[44,45] Patients often present with radial-sided wrist pain and tenderness of the FCR at the level of the trapezium and slightly proximal, which worsens with wrist flexion and radial deviation. Radiographs can be obtained to evaluate for fracture of the scaphoid or trapezium as well as degenerative changes. Advanced imaging is not routinely ordered, but ultrasound and MRI can identify tenosynovitis, tendinopathy, complete and partial tears of the FCR, and local ganglion cysts. Recent literature documents that FCR tendinopathy can be an incidental finding on MRI up to 55% of the time.[44,46] Conservative treatment is similar to other tendinopathies and includes activity modification, immobilization in a wrist and basilar thumb-based splint, anti-inflammatory medications, and therapy for stretching and strengthening. There is a paucity of literature discussing the efficacy and safety of CSIs into the FCR sheath. Lidocaine injection into the sheath can be used, however, for diagnostic confirmation.[47]

In recalcitrant cases, surgical decompression of the FCR tunnel is warranted, with a short period of immobilization postoperatively.[20,42,47] Traditionally, the FCR release is completed through the carpal tunnel where the retinacular septum is opened from inside of the tunnel. Gabel and colleagues[47] reported 10 patients with an average follow-up of 44 months, 9 of whom returned to their previous jobs, with 2 having lifting restrictions. A newer technique, described by Brink and colleagues,[42] uses a minimally invasive and blind technique to tenolyse the FCR tendon. At a median follow-up of 58 months, 26 patients (63%) of 41 were satisfied with the result of the surgery and had no complaints. Ten patients (25%) had less severe or almost the same complaints, and 5 patients (12%) had worsened complaints.

BONE AND JOINT DISORDERS
Ulnocarpal Impaction Syndrome
Ulnocarpal impaction syndrome, also known as ulnar abutment, is caused by repetitive contact of the ulnar head with the TFCC and carpus. It is a degenerative condition that occurs most commonly in patients with positive ulnar variance, because increasing ulnar variance by 2.5 mm can increase the load across the ulnocarpal joint from 16% to 20% to 42%.[48,49] The actions of pronation, ulnar deviation, and power grip, however, dynamically increase ulnar variance, which puts athletes who play baseball and racquet sports at risk.[50] In gymnasts, repetitive loading of the wrist can cause premature closure of the distal radial physis, leading to positive ulnar variance and predisposing the athlete to ulnocarpal abutment.[51] A spectrum of pathology can occur, including degenerative tear of the TFCC; chondromalacia of the lunate, triquetrum, or distal ulna; lunotriquetral ligament tear with possible instability; and distal radioulnar joint osteoarthritis.[5,39,48] Patients have insidious onset of vague ulnar-sided wrist pain that is worsened with wrist loading, pronation, and ulnar deviation. There may be swelling and tenderness at the ulnar fovea, prestyloid recess, lunate, or lunotriquetral articulation. An ulnocarpal stress test can be performed by ulnarly deviating and axially loading the wrist, while moving it through full pronosupination. Reproducible pain with clicking or crepitance is considered a positive maneuver.[52] Plain wrist radiographs of 0° anteroposterior and lateral views can be helpful in identifying ulnar-positive variance, subchondral sclerosis or cysts, or kissing lesions of the lunate, triquetrum, and ulnar head.[49] Pronated power-grip views of the wrist also may help identify dynamic-positive ulnar variance. MRI can be helpful to identify TFCC tears, which usually are central, and signal changes within the lunate, triquetrum, and ulnar head as well as lunotriquetral ligament tears[41] (Fig. 3). Tears of the TFCC are degenerative and can be categorized as class 2 in the Palmer classification system. An in-depth review of TFCC tears is beyond the scope of this article. The gradual progression of this condition allows the athlete to delay any aggressive or invasive treatment until postseason and provides an opportunity for an attempt at nonoperative management. Conservative treatment consists of activity modification and semirigid braces to avoid or block provocative maneuvers while continuing play, rigid immobilization between sporting events, anti-inflammatory medications, and CSIs.[4,53]

If symptoms fail to improve, surgical treatment to correct the positive ulnar variance and débride the central TFCC tear usually is undertaken at a time that is convenient for the athlete. Numerous approaches have been described,

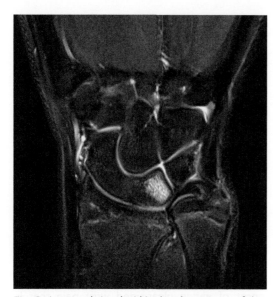

Fig. 3. Increased signal within the ulnar aspect of the lunate as seen with ulnocarpal abutment on a T2-weighted coronal MRI sequence. Also, note the positive ulnar variance.

including open and arthroscopic wafer procedures, ulnar shortening osteotomy (USO), and distal ulnar metaphyseal closing-wedge osteotomy, each with its own advantages and disadvantages. The wafer procedure can be done open or arthroscopically and involves removal of the distal 2 mm to 3 mm of the ulna. This procedure does violate the articular surface and cannot correct ulnar styloid impaction, but, compared with USO, it avoids the known complications of nonunion and implant irritation and has a shorter period of immobilization at only 2 weeks.[53] The USO can be made in various ways at the diaphysis, with an oblique cut or step-cut, and has the advantage of preserving the ulnar articular surface and tightening the extrinsic ligaments. The osteotomy then is fixed with a lag screw and plate, requiring protection in a cast or splint for 4 weeks to 6 weeks postoperatively.[53] There have been reports of up to 50% of patients requiring implant removal after USO.[54] A recent systematic review stated that satisfaction rates were 100% for the arthroscopic wafer procedure, 89% for the open wafer procedure, and 84% for the USO.[55] Additionally, Slade and Gillon described a closing-wedge osteotomy that included removing 5 mm of bone at the articular and metaphyseal junction, which then is stabilized with compression screws; 4 weeks to 6 weeks of postoperative immobilization is required for healing of the

osteotomy site. Patients in their series showed complete recovery and good motion at 2 months.[56]

Ulnar Styloid Impaction Syndrome

Ulnar styloid impaction syndrome (USIS) is a distinct entity that occurs less often than ulnocarpal impaction syndrome. USIS occurs in patients with excessively long ulnar styloids, either as a normal anatomic variant or resulting from a prior trauma with malunion or nonunion of the styloid.[57] The ulnar styloid impacts into the triquetrum, causing pain that is localized to the ulnar side of the wrist. Unlike ulnocarpal abutment, USIS often is seen in ulnar-neutral and ulnar-negative patients. The most likely position to produce impaction and pain is wrist extension and supination, which is a common hand position used when taking slap shots in hockey.[58] Additionally, dynamic impingement has been described in athletes who play golf and racquet sports as well as those with ligamentous laxity.[5] On examination, there is tenderness to palpation of the ulnar styloid, which is volar and deep to the ECU tendon. The examination maneuver, described by Topper and colleagues,[59] involves the placing the hand in standard examining position and with the forearm in neutral rotation. With the wrist fully extended, the forearm is maximally supinated. Reproducible pain is considered a positive maneuver.

USIS is a clinical diagnosis, but radiographs can be confirmatory by demonstrating a decreased distance between the ulnar styloid and triquetrum, ulnar styloid nonunion, sclerosis, flattening of the ulnar styloid, kissing cysts, and loose bodies. MRI can identify bone marrow edema and cystic changes within the ulnar styloid and triquetrum before radiographic changes.[58] Conservative treatments include activity modification, immobilization, anti-inflammatory medications, therapy, and CSIs, which can be both diagnostic and therapeutic. Refractory cases may need a partial or complete ulnar styloid excision, taking care to leave the insertion of the TFCC undisturbed. Patients are placed in a Muenster-type splint for 2 weeks postoperatively, and athletes are instructed to refrain from competitive activities for a total of 6 weeks.[59,60] Literature describing outcomes after styloidectomy is limited, but 1 series of 8 patients reported that 5 were able to return to work without physical restrictions.[59] D'Agostino and colleagues[61] described a novel technique using an oblique ulnar styloid shortening osteotomy to preserve the ligamentous attachments on the styloid. The styloid is fixed with a single

1.5-mm compression screw, and patients are able to initiate range of motion immediately after surgery. All 5 patients had improvement in pain and 4 were able to return to regular activities, but a timeframe was not specified.

Hamatolunate Impaction Syndrome

Approximately 50% of the population has a Viegas type II lunate, in which there is a second facet distally that articulates with the hamate. This anatomic variant can be associated with hamatolunate impaction syndrome and results in chondromalacia and osteoarthritis at this articulation.[62,63] Ulnar deviation alters the biomechanics in the midcarpal row, causing the hamate to articulate with the lunate facet and increasing the load on the proximal hamate.[5] Although it has not been previously documented in the literature, it would seem that athletes participating in golf and racquet sports that require repetitive ulnar deviation would be at risk for developing hamatolunate impaction syndrome. Patients complain of vague ulnar-sided wrist pain. On examination, pain is reproduced with forced ulnar deviation and can be intensified by combining ulnar deviation with a Lichtman test for ulnar midcarpal instability.[64] The Lichtman test consists of a painful click that can be reproduced with axial compression, ulnar deviation, and pronation of the wrist from a neutral position.[65] Radiographs can demonstrate lunate morphology, and images taken in radial and ulnar deviation depict how the hamatolunate articulation is positioned and prone to impingement while in ulnar deviation. Sclerosis, cysts, and degenerative changes also can be visualized. MRI shows bone marrow edema, cartilage defects, sclerosis, and subchondral cysts.[66] Conservative treatment can be attempted while an athlete continues competing and consists of immobilization, anti-inflammatory medications, and CSIs. Surgical intervention can be undertaken at a time convenient for the athlete and may include open excision of the head of the hamate or arthroscopic burring of the hamate. A report of 4 nonathlete patients reported that all had improvement in their pain and returned to previous activities postoperatively.[64]

Dorsal Wrist Impingement Syndromes

Athletes who subject their wrists to repetitive extension, especially in combination with axial loading, are predisposed to development of dorsal wrist impingement syndromes (DWISs).[51] Notably, gymnasts are at risk, but athletes who participate in platform diving and shot put also load their wrists in a hyperextended position.[51,67] Numerous theories have been proposed to explain DWISs, and some surgeons even question their existence as a discrete diagnosis. Henry[68] classified primary DWIS as simply a capsular impingement between ECRB and the scaphoid. He described secondary DWIS as caused by scapholunate instability or rotatory subluxation of the scaphoid that causes a dorsal shift of the proximal pole, exaggerating the same mechanism of capsular impingement.[68]

The spectrum of DWISs involving rotatory subluxation of the scaphoid was first described by Watson and colleagues,[69] who also believed this to be an underlying cause of dorsal wrist ganglion cysts.[70] Additionally, Terng and colleagues[71] found entrapment of subcapsular fibrous tissue in the radiocarpal and intercarpal joints to be a common source of dorsal wrist pain. Lastly, impingement of the extensor retinaculum has also been described.[67] All these processes can lead to dorsal capsular thickening with capsulitis, synovitis, and development of dorsal wrist ganglia. The etiology may involve acute trauma or repetitive microtrauma. Patients describe exacerbation of dorsal wrist pain when in the push-up position. There are no specific examination maneuvers for DWISs, so an examination should be thorough, documenting swelling, tenderness to palpation, range of motion, a scaphoid shift test, and a resisted extension test. Pain with terminal extension and dorsal radiocarpal tenderness are common findings.[72] The diagnosis is made clinically, but radiographs and MRI can be used to rule out other sources of pain such as fracture, ligamentous pathology, osteonecrosis, and degenerative changes.[51] In chronic cases, radiographs can show dorsal osteophytes of the distal radial rim, scaphoid, and lunate.[2] Most patient's symptoms resolve with a course of conservative treatment, lasting weeks to months, that centers around avoidance of loading the wrist in extension. This can be accomplished with rest or limiting the provocative maneuver with use of braces when competing. Other nonoperative treatments include anti-inflammatory medications and CSIs.[5,51,72]

Surgical treatments are available for refractory cases and can be performed at a time convenient for the athlete. Open treatments include dorsal capsulectomy, débridement of dorsal bony ridges on the scaphoid and lunate, and posterior interosseous nerve neurectomy.[69,70] Arthroscopic treatments include synovectomy with complete capsulectomy to visualize the ECRB tendon and partial capsulectomy of only the redundant capsule.[68,72,73]

Patients are placed in soft dressings and range of motion is encouraged immediately after all the variants of surgery, discussed previously. Although there is no literature reporting outcomes in athletes, Matson and colleagues[72] showed significant improvement in pain and functional outcomes at 1-month clinical follow-up and 41-month telephone follow-up. Yasuda and colleagues[70] reported that 17 of 20 patients were pain-free or had mild pain at 37 months after surgery. Occult dorsal wrist ganglia also may occur with DWISs and should be resected with an open or arthroscopic approach at the time of any surgical intervention.

DISTAL RADIAL PHYSEAL INJURY

In gymnastics, the wrist is subject to various stresses unique to the sport, including repetitive motion, high-impact loading, axial compression, torsional forces, and distraction in varying degrees of ulnar and radial deviation and hyperextension.[74] Furthermore, the forces across the wrist in different exercises can be up to 16 times the body weight, predisposing the gymnast to several wrist pathologies.[75] Distal radial physeal injury, also called gymnast's wrist or distal radial epiphysitis, is an overuse syndrome seen in skeletally immature gymnasts and is caused by repetitive stress on the distal radial physis. Skeletally immature wrists tend to be more ulnar negative, placing a higher load on the radius. Furthermore, an open physis is more prone to injury because the joint capsule and ligamentous structures are stronger than the cartilaginous physis.[51,76] Repetitive forces to the physis result in a compromised blood supply with widening, microfractures, and a Salter-Harris type I injury. With chronic injury, there can be premature physeal closure resulting in growth arrest.[77-79] In growing children and adolescents who have premature physeal closure of the distal radius, the ulna continues to elongate, resulting in an ulnar-positive wrist and leading to further issues with altered loading of the wrist and the sequelae of ulnocarpal impingement. Additionally, partial physeal closure can result in a Madelung-type deformity of the distal radius.[80] Patients experience pain at the onset of activity that worsens with continued activity. Examination demonstrates tenderness at the distal radial physis and pain reproduced with maximal extension and axial loading.[81] Radiographs can be normal or show a widened physis, specifically at the radial and volar borders, with cystic changes and irregular borders.[41] MRI can show paraphyseal edema and/or physeal bridging,

and recent studies have used advanced imaging to calculate volumes of the widened physis to determine at-risk athletes and to correlate with the severity of physeal stress.[82]

Treatment focuses on the cessation of the inciting activity, and a minimum of 6 weeks' rest typically is required to see symptomatic improvement. Radiographic improvement of physeal changes takes longer, so it is recommended to follow these patients with images at 6 months and 1 year after presentation and initiation of treatment.[51] After clinical resolution of symptoms, the patient can gradually return to weight-bearing activities and consider the use of wrist guards to prevent extreme wrist extension when competing.[74] Surgical treatment is reserved for patients who have premature physeal closure. A partial distal radial physeal closure may warrant resection of the physeal bridge versus completion distal radial epiphysiodesis in conjunction with distal ulnar epiphysiodesis.[83] Ulnar positive wrists with ulnocarpal impingement are treated, as described previously.

SUMMARY

Chronic wrist pain is a sport-specific complaint in athletes and can be caused by a variety of overuse injuries involving tendons, bones, joints, and other soft tissues. Diagnosis usually can be made from a thorough examination and confirmed by a combination of radiographs, ultrasound, and MRI. Most athletes have resolution of symptoms with conservative treatment, but there is evidence to support good functional outcomes and return to play if surgical intervention is required.

CLINICS CARE POINTS

- Overuse injuries of the wrist can occur in athletes of any competitive level, and a detailed history and examination is vital in making a correct diagnosis.
- Specific motions and maneuvers related to individual sports can make athletes more prone to certain injuries.
- In many overuse wrist injuries, a trial of conservative treatment can be attempted before obtaining advanced imaging.
- Various surgical options with favorable outcomes are available for treatment of overuse injuries if conservative treatments are unsuccessful. However, most athletes can be treated successfully

and return to play with conservative measures only.

- A specific treatment plan should be tailored to each athlete, and factors to consider include level of competition, timing during season of play, and length of recovery.

DISCLOSURE

Neither the author nor her immediate family received any financial payments or other benefits from any commercial entity related to the subject of this article.

REFERENCES

1. Amadio P. Epidemiology of hand and wrist injuries in sports. Hand Clin 1990;6:379–81.

2. Amadio P. Epidemiology of hand and wrist injuries in sports. Hand Clin 1990;6:379–81.

3. Geissler W. Ligamentous sports injuries of the hand and wrist. Sports Med Arthrosc Rev 2014;22(1):39–44.

4. Avery DM, Rodner CM, Edgar CM. Sports-related wrist and hand injuries: a review. J Orthop Surg 2016;11(1):99.

5. Llopis E, Restrepo R, Kassarjian A, et al. Overuse injuries of the wrist. Radiol Clin North Am 2019;57(5):957–76.

6. Tagliafico AS, Ameri P, Michaud J, et al. Wrist injuries in nonprofessional tennis players: relationships with different grips. Am J Sports Med 2009;37(4):760–7.

7. Woo S-H, Lee Y-K, Kim J-M, et al. Hand and wrist injuries in golfers and their treatment. Hand Clin 2017;33(1):81–96.

8. Thornton JS, Vinther A, Wilson F, et al. Rowing injuries: an updated review. Sports Med 2017;47(4):641–61.

9. Rossi C, Cellocco P, Margaritondo E, et al. De Quervain disease in volleyball players. Am J Sports Med 2005;33(3):424–7.

10. Clarke MT, Lyall HA, Grant JW, et al. The histopathology of De Quervain's disease. J Hand Surg 1998;23(6):732–4.

11. Adams JE, Habbu R. Tendinopathies of the hand and wrist. J Am Acad Orthop Surg 2015;23(12):741–50.

12. Elliott BG. Finkelstein's test: a descriptive error that can produce a false positive. J Hand Surg 1992;17(4):481–2.

13. Goubau JF, Goubau L, Van Tongel A, et al. The wrist hyperflexion and abduction of the thumb (WHAT) test: a more specific and sensitive test to diagnose de Quervain tenosynovitis than the Eichhoff's test. J Hand Surg Eur Vol 2014;39(3):286–92.

14. McBain B, Rio E, Cook J, et al. Diagnostic accuracy of imaging modalities in the detection of clinically diagnosed de Quervain's syndrome: a systematic review. Skeletal Radiol 2019;48(11):1715–21.

15. Rowland P, Phelan N, Gardiner S, et al. The effectiveness of corticosteroid injection for de Quervain's stenosing tenosynovitis (DQST): a systematic review and meta-analysis. Open Orthop J 2015;9(1):437–44.

16. Ashraf MO, Devadoss VG. Systematic review and meta-analysis on steroid injection therapy for de Quervain's tenosynovitis in adults. Eur J Orthop Surg Traumatol 2014;24(2):149–57.

17. Oh JK, Messing S, Hyrien O, et al. Effectiveness of corticosteroid injections for treatment of de Quervain's tenosynovitis. Hand 2017;12(4):357–61.

18. Ippolito JA, Hauser S, Patel J, et al. Nonsurgical treatment of de Quervain tenosynovitis: a prospective randomized trial. Hand 2020;15(2):215–9.

19. Ilyas AM, Ast M, Schaffer AA, et al. de Quervain tenosynovitis of the wrist. J Am Acad Orthop Surg 2007;15(12):757–64.

20. Patrick NC, Hammert WC. Hand and wrist tendinopathies. Clin Sports Med 2020;39(2):247–58.

21. Kang HJ, Koh IH, Jang JW, et al. Endoscopic versus open release in patients with de Quervain's tenosynovitis: A randomised trial. Bone Joint J 2013;95-B(7):947–51.

22. Grundberg AB, Reagan DS. Pathologic anatomy of the forearm: Intersection syndrome. J Hand Surg 1985;10(2):299–302.

23. Sato J, Ishii Y, Noguchi H. Clinical and ultrasound features in patients with intersection syndrome or de Quervain's disease. J Hand Surg Eur Vol 2016;41(2):220–5.

24. Draghi F, Bortolotto C. Intersection syndrome: ultrasound imaging. Skeletal Radiol 2014;43(3):283–7.

25. Lee RP, Hatem SF, Recht MP. Extended MRI findings of intersection syndrome. Skeletal Radiol 2009;38(2):157–63.

26. Marcus Fulcher S, Kiefhaber TR, Stern PJ. Upper-extremity tendinitis and overuse syndromes in the athlete. Clin Sports Med 1998;17(3):433–48.

27. Hoy G, Trease L, Braybon W. Intersection syndrome: an acute surgical disease in elite rowers. BMJ Open Sport Exerc Med 2019;5(1):e000535.

28. Allende C, Le Viet D. Extensor carpi ulnaris problems at the wrist—classification, surgical treatment and results. J Hand Surg 2005;30(3):265–72.

29. Montalvan B. Extensor carpi ulnaris injuries in tennis players: a study of 28 cases. Commentary. Br J Sports Med 2006;40(5):424–9.

30. McAuliffe JA. Tendon disorders of the hand and wrist. J Hand Surg 2010;35(5):846–53.

31. Carneiro RS, Fontana R, Mazzer N. Ulnar wrist pain in athletes caused by erosion of the floor of the sixth dorsal compartment: a case series. Am J Sports Med 2005;33(12):1910–3.

32. Ruland RT, Hogan CJ. The ECU synergy test: an aid to diagnose ECU tendonitis. J Hand Surg 2008; 33(10):1777–82.

33. Sato J, Ishii Y, Noguchi H. Diagnostic performance of the extensor carpi ulnaris (ECU) synergy test to detect sonographic ecu abnormalities in chronic dorsal ulnar-sided wrist pain. J Ultrasound Med 2016;35(1):7–14.

34. Jeantroux J, Becce F, Guerini H, et al. Athletic injuries of the extensor carpi ulnaris subsheath: MRI findings and utility of gadolinium-enhanced fat-saturated T1-weighted sequences with wrist pronation and supination. Eur Radiol 2011;21(1):160–6.

35. Campbell D, Campbell R, O'Connor P, al at. Sports-related extensor carpi ulnaris pathology: a review of functional anatomy, sports injury and management. Br J Sports Med 2013;47(17): 1105–11.

36. Patterson SM, Picconatto WJ, Alexander JA, et al. Conservative treatment of an acute traumatic extensor carpi ulnaris tendon subluxation in a collegiate basketball player: a case report. J Athl Train 2011;46(5):574–6.

37. Puri SK, Morse KW, Hearns KA, et al. A biomechanical comparison of extensor carpi ulnaris subsheath reconstruction techniques. J Hand Surg 2017;42(10):837.e1–7.

38. Graham TJ. Pathologies of the extensor carpi ulnaris (ECU) tendon and its investments in the athlete. Hand Clin 2012;28(3):345–56.

39. Dineen HA, Greenberg JA. Ulnar-sided wrist pain in the athlete. Clin Sports Med 2020;39(2):373–400.

40. Budoff JE, Kraushaar BS, Ayala G. Flexor carpi ulnaris tendinopathy. J Hand Surg 2005;30(1):125–9.

41. Cockenpot E, Lefebvre G, Demondion X, et al. Imaging of sports-related hand and wrist injuries: sports imaging series. Radiology 2016;279(3): 674–92.

42. Brink PRG, Franssen BBGM, Disseldorp DJG. A simple blind tenolysis for flexor carpi radialis tendinopathy. Hand 2015;10(2):323–7.

43. Bishop AT, Gabel G, Carmichael SW. Flexor carpi radialis tendinitis, Part I: Operative anatomy. J Bone Joint Surg 1994;76A:1009–14.

44. Stoop N, van der Gronde BATD, Janssen SJ, et al. Incidental flexor carpi radialis tendinopathy on magnetic resonance imaging. Hand 2019;14(5):632–5.

45. Parellada AJ, Morrison WB, Reiter SB, et al. Flexor carpi radialis tendinopathy: spectrum of imaging findings and association with triscaphe arthritis. Skeletal Radiol 2006;35(8):572–8.

46. Luong D, Smith J, Bianchi S. Flexor carpi radialis tendon ultrasound pictoral essay. Skeletal Radiol 2014;43(6):745–60.

47. Gabel G, Bishop AT, Wood MB. Flexor carpi radialis tendinitis. Part ii: Results of operative treatment. J Bone Joint Surg 1994;76A:1015–8.

48. Friedman SL, Palmer AK. The ulnar impaction syndrome. Hand Clin 1991;7(2):295–310.

49. Sachar K. Ulnar-sided wrist pain: evaluation and treatment of triangular fibrocartilage complex tears, ulnocarpal impaction syndrome, and lunotriquetral ligament tears. J Hand Surg 2012;37(7): 1489–500.

50. Friedman SL, Palmer AK, Short WH, et al. The change in ulnar variance with grip. J Hand Surg 1993;18(4):713–6.

51. Benjamin HJ, Engel SC, Chudzik D. Wrist pain in gymnasts: a review of common overuse wrist pathology in the gymnastics athlete. Curr Sports Med Rep 2017;16(5):322–9.

52. Nakamura R, Horii E, Imaeda T, et al. The ulnocarpal stress test in the diagnosis of ulnar-sided wrist pain. J Hand Surg Br 1997;22(6):719–23.

53. Jarrett CD, Baratz ME. The management of ulnocarpal abutment and degenerative triangular fibrocartilage complex tears in the competitive athlete. Hand Clin 2012;28(3):329–37.

54. Bernstein MA, Nagle DJ, Martinez A, et al. A comparison of combined arthroscopic triangular fibrocartilage complex debridement and arthroscopic wafer distal ulna resection versus arthroscopic triangular fibrocartilage complex debridement and ulnar shortening osteotomy for ulnocarpal abutment syndrome. Arthroscopy 2004;20(4):392–401.

55. Stockton DJ, Pelletier M-E, Pike JM. Operative treatment of ulnar impaction syndrome: a systematic review. J Hand Surg Eur Vol 2015;40(5): 470–6.

56. Slade JF, Gillon TJ. Osteochondral shortening osteotomy for the treatment of ulnar impaction syndrome: a new technique. Tech Hand Up Extrem Surg 2007;11(1):9.

57. Watanabe A, Souza F, Vezeridis PS, et al. Ulnar-sided wrist pain. II. Clinical imaging and treatment. Skeletal Radiol 2010;39(9):837–57.

58. Giachino AA, McIntyre AI, Guy KJ, et al. Ulnar styloid triquetral impaction. Hand Surg 2007;12(02): 123–34.

59. Topper SM, Wood MB, Ruby LK. Ulnar styloid impaction syndrome. J Hand Surg 1997;22(4): 699–704.

60. Tomaino MM, Gainer M, Towers JD. Carpal impaction with the ulnar styloid process: treatment with partial styloid resection. J Hand Surg 2001;26(3): 252–5.

61. D'Agostino P, Townley WA, Le Viet D, et al. Oblique ulnar styloid osteotomy—a treatment for ulnar styloid impaction syndrome. J Hand Surg 2011; 36(11):1785–9.

62. Viegas SF, Wagner K, Patterson R, et al. Medial (hamate) facet of the lunate. J Hand Surg 1990; 15(4):564–71.

63. Malik AM, Schweitzer ME, Culp RW, et al. MR imaging of the type II lunate bone: frequency, extent, and associated findings. Am J Roentgenol 1999; 173(2):335–8.

64. Thurston AJ, Stanley JK. Hamato-lunate impingement: An uncommon cause of ulnar-sided wrist pain. Arthroscopy 2000;16(5):540–4.

65. Lichtman DM, Schneider JR, Swafford AR, et al. Ulnar midcarpal instability—Clinical and laboratory analysis. J Hand Surg 1981;6(5):515–23.

66. Pfirrmann C, Theumann N, Chung C, et al. The hamatolunate facet: characterization and association with cartilage lesions – magnetic resonance arthrography and anatomic correlation in cadaveric wrists. Skeletal Radiol 2002;31(8):451–6.

67. VanHeest AE, Luger NM, House JH, et al. Extensor retinaculum impingement in the athlete: a new diagnosis. Am J Sports Med 2007;35(12): 2126–30.

68. Henry M. Arthroscopic management of dorsal wrist impingement. J Hand Surg 2008;33(7):1201–4.

69. Watson KH, Rogers WD, Ashmead D. Reevaluation of the cause of the wrist ganglion. J Hand Surg 1989;14(5):812–7.

70. Yasuda M, Masada K, Takeuchi E. Dorsal wrist syndrome repair. Hand Surg 2004;09(01):45–8.

71. Terng SCA, Kuypers KC, Koch AR. Inter-carpal soft tissue entrapment. a possible explanation for chronic dorsal wrist pain. J Hand Surg 2006;31(1): 41–6.

72. Matson AP, Dekker TJ, Lampley AJ, et al. Diagnosis and arthroscopic management of dorsal wrist capsular impingement. J Hand Surg 2017;42(3): e167–74.

73. Jain K, Singh R. Short-term result of arthroscopic synovial excision for dorsal wrist pain in hyperextension associated with synovial hypertrophy. Singapore Med J 2014;55(10):547–9.

74. Webb BG, Rettig LA. Gymnastic wrist injuries. Curr Sports Med Rep 2008;7(5):289–95.

75. Markolf KL, Shapiro MS, Mandelbaum BR, et al. Wrist loading patterns during pommel horse exercises. J Biomech 1990;23(10):1001–11.

76. Poletto ED, Pollock AN. Radial epiphysitis (aka gymnast wrist). Pediatr Emerg Care 2012;28(5):484–5.

77. DiFiori JP, Puffer JC, Aish B, et al. Wrist pain, distal radial physeal injury, and ulnar variance in young gymnasts: does a relationship exist? Am J Sports Med 2002;30(6):879–85.

78. Bancroft LW. Wrist injuries. Radiol Clin North Am 2013;51(2):299–311.

79. Wolf MR, Avery D, Wolf JM. Upper extremity injuries in gymnasts. Hand Clin 2017;33(1):187–97.

80. Vender MI, Kirk Watson H. Acquired Madelung-like deformity in a gymnast. J Hand Surg 1988;13(1): 19–21.

81. Ashwell ZR, Richardson ML. Gymnast's wrist in a 12-year-old female with MRI correlation. Radiol Case Rep 2019;14(3):360–4.

82. Kraan RBJ, Kox LS, Mens MA, et al. Damage of the distal radial physis in young gymnasts: can three-dimensional assessment of physeal volume on MRI serve as a biomarker? Eur Radiol 2019;29(11): 6364–71.

83. Paz DA, Chang GH, Yetto JM, et al. Upper extremity overuse injuries in pediatric athletes: clinical presentation, imaging findings, and treatment. Clin Imaging 2015;39(6):954–64.

Scaphoid Fractures in Athletes

William J. Weller, MD[1], Norfleet B. Thompson, MD*, Sierra G. Phillips, MD[1], James H. Calandruccio, MD[1]

KEYWORDS

• Scaphoid fracture • Athletes • Percutaneous fixation • Open reduction • Return to play

KEY POINTS

- The scaphoid is the most commonly injured carpal bone in athletes.
- Most fractures can be treated with cast immobilization, with an expected rate of union of 90% to 95%.
- Operative treatment typically is recommended for unstable fractures in which the fragments are offset more than 1 mm.
- Fixation can be obtained with percutaneous or open techniques.
- Closed reduction and percutaneous screw fixation generally are preferred in athletes to allow a quicker return to sport.

The scaphoid is the most commonly injured carpal bone in athletes,[1,2] with a high incidence in college football players and an increasing incidence in female athletes.[3] Scaphoid fractures account for 50% to 80% of all carpal bone fractures in young and active individuals.[4] The typical mechanism of injury is wrist hyperextension with the hand pronated and radially deviated (Fig. 1). The scaphoid usually fractures in tension with the wrist extended, concentrating the load on the radial-palmar side.

DIAGNOSIS

Presentation can range from disabling wrist pain to mild swelling and decreased range of motion. It is not uncommon to find a scaphoid nonunion with a remote history of a wrist sprain. Athletes usually complain of radial-sided wrist pain with exquisite tenderness in the anatomic snuff box (Fig. 2) and pain with axial loading of the thumb or with pincer grasp. Radiographic assessment of the wrist should include posteroanterior (PA), lateral, and ulnar-deviated views. Because of subtle fracture lines and the irregular contour of the scaphoid, nondisplaced fractures can be missed on radiographs, and advanced imaging with computed tomography (CT) is needed for fracture identification or alignment. MRI or bone scintigraphy may be needed to confirm the diagnosis. A Cochrane review article comparing CT, MRI, and bone scintigraphy for the diagnosis of occult scaphoid fractures found that bone scintigraphy was the most sensitive test (0.99) compared with CT (0.72) and MRI (0.88), but was less specific (0.86) than either CT (0.99) or MRI (1.00). Bone scintigraphy also requires a 72-hour delay from injury, is more invasive, and is not recommended in children because of radiation exposure. CT and MRI are both useful, with CT providing better information about fracture configuration if needed for preoperative planning.[5]

CLASSIFICATION

There have been several classification systems described for scaphoid fractures, including those proposed by Cooney and colleagues, Russe, Prosser, and OTA.[6,7] For many years, the

Department of Orthopaedic Surgery & Biomechanical Engineering, University of Tennessee-Campbell Clinic, Memphis, TN, USA
[1]Present address: 1400 South Germantown Road, Germantown, TN 38138.
* Corresponding author. Campbell Clinic, 1400 South Germantown Road, Germantown, TN 38138.
E-mail address: nbthompson@campbellclinic.com

Orthop Clin N Am 51 (2020) 511–516
https://doi.org/10.1016/j.ocl.2020.07.001
0030-5898/20/© 2020 Elsevier Inc. All rights reserved.

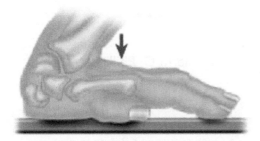

Fig. 1. Mechanism of injury of scaphoid fractures. The arrow simply refers to the "axial load" associated with scaphoid fractures.

Herbert classification has been the most used system[8]; however, the interobserver reliability of the Herbert system is rated as only fair.[9] Most classification systems are based on fracture location, displacement, or stability as determined on radiographs. Buijze and colleagues[9] in a prospective arthroscopic study challenged the ability to accurately predict stability based on static radiographs or CT. In a recent Instructional Course Lecture, Buijze and colleagues[10] recommended a simple descriptive classification based on fracture location (eg, proximal third) and the magnitude and nature of displacement (eg, minimally displaced <1 mm) as the most useful. The system described by Cooney and colleagues is a simple classification of scaphoid fractures as either undisplaced and stable or displaced and unstable.[11] A scaphoid fracture is classified as displaced (unstable) if radiographs show more than 1 mm of displacement on anterior-posterior and oblique radiographic views, more than 15° of lunocapitate angulation on a lateral view, or more than 45° of scapholunate angulation on a lateral view. Because the ranges of lunocapitate and scapholunate

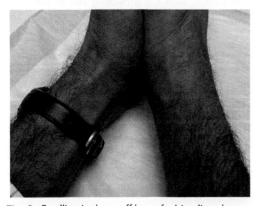

Fig. 2. Swelling in the snuff box of a bicyclist who sustained a scaphoid fracture. (*From* Belsky MR, Leibman MI, Ruchelsman DE. Scaphoid fracture in the elite athlete. Hand Clin 2012; 28:269-278.)

angulation can vary, comparison views of the opposite wrist can be helpful.

TREATMENT

Reduction can be attempted initially by longitudinal traction and slight radial compression of the carpus. Nonoperative treatment usually is successful for acute nondisplaced, stable fractures without other bony or ligamentous injury. With nonoperative casting techniques, the expected rate of union is 90% to 95% within 10 to 12 weeks. Fractures at and distal to the scaphoid waist are expected to heal sooner than those in the proximal pole. During this time, the fracture is observed radiographically for healing. Some athletes may be able to use padded casts during competition.[12] Cast treatment, however, has the disadvantages of longer immobilization time, joint stiffness, reduced grip strength, and longer time to return to manual work or athletics.

If collapse or angulation of the fractured fragments occurs, surgical treatment usually is required. Surgery also should be considered if new healing activity is not evident and if union is not apparent after a trial of cast immobilization for about 20 weeks. Most minimally displaced scaphoid fractures and all displaced scaphoid fractures in elite athletes are treated with early fixation to maximally expedite the return to full function.

Operative treatment typically is recommended for an unstable fracture in which the fragments are offset more than 1 mm in the anteroposterior or oblique view (**Fig. 3**), or lunocapitate angulation is greater than 15°, or the scapholunate angulation is greater than 45° in the lateral view (range 30°–60°). Other criteria for evaluating displacement include a lateral intrascaphoid angle greater than 45°, an anteroposterior intrascaphoid angle less than 35°, and a height-to-length ratio of 0.65 or greater. If closed reduction is successful, percutaneous fixation with a cannulated screw or pins and application of a thumb spica cast may suffice. Otherwise, open reduction and internal fixation may be required.

Percutaneous Screw Fixation

Percutaneous fixation is aimed at reducing damage to the blood supply and soft tissues, allowing early mobilization of the wrist and early return to sports. The best available evidence for percutaneous screw fixation versus cast treatment suggests that percutaneous fixation allows a faster time to union by 5 weeks.[13] Goffin and

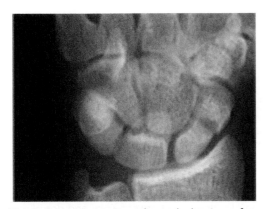

Fig. 3. Posterior-anterior radiograph showing a fracture of the scaphoid with a 1 mm gap and step. (*From* Dias JJ, Singh HP. Displaced fracture of the waist of the scaphoid. J Bone Joint Surg Br 2011; 93-B:1433-1439.)

colleagues,[14] in their meta-analysis comparing outcomes of conservative treatment and operative treatment (eg, percutaneous screw fixation, open reduction, and internal fixation), found significantly better union rates and better return-to-sports rates with operative treatment. With conservative treatment, the return-to-sport rate was 90%, and average time to return to sport was 9.6 weeks; with operative treatment, the return-to-sport rate was 98%, and average time to return to sport was 7.3 weeks. Prospective, randomized studies comparing percutaneous screw fixation with cast immobilization also have showed that patients with screw fixation were able to regain movement and return to most activities earlier than patients treated with casting. In a prospective randomized study of nondisplaced scaphoid waist fractures, there were no nonunions in the 44 patients treated with screw fixation without postoperative immobilization, but 10 nonunions were present at 12 weeks in the 44 patients treated with cast immobilization.[15] Cited advantages of limited access, percutaneous, and arthroscopic percutaneous fixation include less risk to neurovascular structures and intercarpal ligaments, earlier bone healing, and earlier return to activities. In their meta-analysis, however, Ibrahim and colleagues[16] noted a significantly increased complication rate with operative treatment, and Bushnell and colleagues[17] suggested that complications of dorsal percutaneous cannulated screw fixation may be more common than previously reported. In Bushnell and colleagues study of 24 patients with percutaneous screw fixation, they noted complications in 29%, including nonunion, implant problems, and postoperative fracture.

Percutaneous screws can be inserted through a volar (**Fig. 4**A) or dorsal (**Fig. 4**B) approach. Although there are proponents for each approach, studies have found little or no difference in outcomes or complications. In a meta-analysis, Kang and colleagues[18] found similar outcomes in union rates, complications, overall functional outcome, postoperative pain, grip strength, flexion, extension, and radial deviation; ulnar deviation, however, was significantly greater with the volar approach. Biomechanical studies have reported that central screw placement is related to biomechanically superior outcomes.[19–21] Although central screw position can be more reliably achieved using a dorsal approach, it is unclear whether these biomechanical advantages are accompanied by clinical advantages. Kang and colleagues[18] concluded that the results of their meta-analysis did not support the theoretic advantage of the dorsal approach over the volar approach, because all but one of the tested parameters, including nonunion rate, among the most important parameters for assessing the clinical outcomes of fracture treatment, did not differ between the 2 approaches.

Dodds and colleagues[22] described a simple, dorsal, miniopen approach to the scaphoid that minimizes incision size, extensor tendon dissection, capsular trauma, and vascular disruption, while still allowing direct visualization of the proximal pole and optimal exposure for accurate screw placement. In their study comparing the mini-open approach to a dorsal percutaneous approach, they found no significant difference in complication rates. Verstreken and colleagues[23] described a transtrapezial technique that they characterized as technically easier than conventional techniques of percutaneous scaphoid fixation and associated with a lower risk of complications. This technique does not require manipulation of the wrist or scaphoid to insert the guidewire. Additionally, it provides access to the central axis of the scaphoid; less fluoroscopy time is needed, and there is less risk of soft-tissue damage around the scaphoid. With exact central placement of the screw providing rigid fixation, no formal immobilization is necessary, and early return to activity is allowed. In 41 patients in whom this approach was used, all fractures healed within 10 weeks, and functional ranges of wrist motion and grip strength were achieved in all patients. At 3-year follow-up, radiographs showed accurate central placement of the screw in all patients, and no degenerative changes were seen at the scaphotrapezial joint.

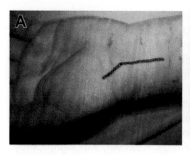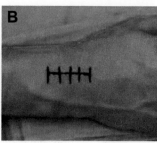

Fig. 4. Approaches for percutaneous fixation. (*A*) Volar approach. (*B*) Dorsal approach. (*From* Yam H. Scaphoid fractures and HCS. SlideShare, published on May 28, 2019.)

ARTHROSCOPY

Arthroscopy has been suggested for determining the alignment of the reduced scaphoid and assessing adjacent injuries to the ligaments and other carpal bones.[24,25] Arthroscopy also is useful, because it allows control of the fracture reduction and evaluation of screw protrusion.[26] When CT imaging does not clearly demonstrate whether a scaphoid fracture has united, arthroscopic wrist surgery can be used to obtain additional information to determine whether the fracture has united, partially united, or has not united. Slade and colleagues, however, warned that percutaneous arthroscopic fixation is associated with a steep learning curve. Complications include intraoperative breakage of the equipment such as the screw and guide wires, and eccentric placement of the screw or its being too long. The screw may protrude into the joint, or, as it is advanced, impact against the opposite cortex, causing distraction of the fracture. Eccentric placement may lead to poor stability, and dorsal tendons can be damaged by percutaneous wires.[27] Currently, there is no published evidence that arthroscopic assistance improves the outcome of the treatment of scaphoid fractures.

Open Reduction and Internal Fixation

Open treatment of scaphoid fractures is typically recommended for fractures that are displaced greater than 1 mm or are unstable, comminuted, malreduced (humpback deformity), or irreducible by closed or percutaneous methods. Two meta-analyses have advocated an open approach to scaphoid fracture management over closed and percutaneous treatments.[28,29] Open reduction can be done through a volar or dorsal approach (**Fig. 5**), both of which provide improved visualization of the fracture and confirmation of an anatomic reduction before headless compression screw placement. Reports have demonstrated equal success and complication rates between volar and dorsal approaches. The dorsal approach is typically advocated for proximal scaphoid fractures and nonunions for improved central axis placement of a single headless compression screw. Disadvantages of the dorsal approach include inferior visualization of the fracture compared with the volar approach, potential for fracture displacement and iatrogenic humpback deformity that occurs with wrist hyperflexion that is required during screw insertion, and damage to the dorsal blood supply. The volar approach to the scaphoid is most often used for distal third fractures and for correction of a flexed scaphoid deformity. The entire volar surface of the scaphoid can be visualized, allowing for reduction confirmation that is particularly useful in cases of volar bone loss, comminution, or the need to correct a scaphoid humpback deformity. Disadvantages of the volar approach include damage to the scaphotrapezial joint to obtain an appropriate trajectory and potential injury to the volar wrist-stabilizing structures.[30]

RETURN TO ACTIVITY

Return to activity depends on the patient characteristics and the type of the fracture; thus, the decision on when to resume normal activities should be personalized to each patient. Brekke and colleagues[31] noted that inherent stability of the scaphoid was maintained with at least 25% scaphoid waist intact. Most, however, prefer to have evidence of union in 50% of the fracture and evidence of a firmly seated screw. The risk of refracture is high, and patients generally are advised to refrain from participating in contact sports for 2 to 3 months following healing; this can be especially challenging in competitive athletes. Some athletes can use playing casts, which are generally softer and lighter, during games to protect both the patient and other players from injury. Soft casts were not found to influence the outcome or delay healing.[32]

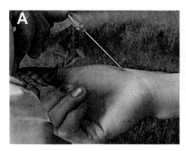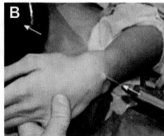

Fig. 5. Open approaches. (*A*) Volar approach. (*B*) Dorsal approach. (*From* Milton R. Scaphoid fractures and non union. SlideShare, published on February 1, 2017.)

Competitive athletes and sports players whose careers are at stake usually are allowed to return to play as soon as it is safely possible.

SUMMARY

Scaphoid fractures are common injuries in athletes. Most can be treated with cast immobilization, with an expected rate of union of 90% to 95%. Cast treatment, however, has the disadvantages of longer immobilization time, joint stiffness, reduced grip strength, and longer time to return to manual work or athletics. Closed reduction and percutaneous screw fixation generally are preferred in athletes to allow a quicker return to sport; if closed reduction cannot be obtained, open reduction and internal fixation may be required.

CLINICS CARE POINTS

- A high index of suspicion for scaphoid fractures is warranted in treating acute wrist injuries in athletes.
- Successful fracture fixation results in earlier return to play for athletes.
- Operative approach should be dictated by the fracture location and geometry. Proximal pole fractures are approached dorsally. More distal fractures especially those with humpback deformity are approached volarly.
- Percutaneous methods may be used for minimally displaced fractures to achieve faster union.

DISCLOSURE

The authors have nothing to disclose.

REFERENCES

1. Liu EH, Alqahtani S, Alsaaran RN, et al. A prospective study of pediatric hand fractures and review of the literature. Pediatr Emerg Care 2014;30(5):299–304.
2. Caine D, Purcell L. Injury in pediatric and adolescent sports: epidemiology, treatment and prevention. Cham (Switzerland): Springer; 2016.
3. Swenson DM, Henke NM, Collins CL, et al. Epidemiology of United States high school sports-related fractures, 2008-09 to 2010-11. Am J Sports Med 2012;40(9):2078–84.
4. Mallee WH, Wang J, Poolman RW, et al. Computed tomography vs magnetic resonance imaging vs bone scintigraphy for clinically suspected scaphoid fractures in patients with negative plain radiographs. Cochrane Database Syst Rev 2015;2015(6): CD10023.
5. Majeed H. Non-operative treatment versus percutaneous fixation of minimally displaced scaphoid waist fractures in high demand young manual workers. J Orthop Trauma 2014;15:239–44.
6. Marsh JL, Slongo TF, Agel J, et al. Fracture and dislocation classification compendium – 2007; Orthopaedic Trauma Association Classification, Database, and Outcomes Committee. J Orthop Trauma 2007;21(10 Suppl):S1–133.
7. Prosser AJ, Brenkel IJ, Irvine GB. Articular fractures of the distal scaphoid. J Hand Surg Br 1988;13: 87–91.
8. Ten Berg PW, Drijkoningen T, Strackee SD, et al. Classifications of acute scaphoid fractures: a systematic literature review. J Wrist Surg 2016;5(2):152–9.
9. Buijze GA, Jørgsholm P, Thomsen NO, et al. Diagnostic performance of radiographs and computed tomography for displacement and instability of acute scaphoid waist fractures. J Bone Joint Surg Am 2012;94(21):1967–74.
10. Buijze GA, Bachoura A, Mahmood B, et al. Revaluation of the scaphoid fracture: what is the best current evidence? Instr Course Lect 2020;69:317–30.
11. Cooney WP, Dobyns JH, Linscheid RL. Fractures of the scaphoid: a rational approach to management. Clin Orthop Relat Res 1980;149:90–7.
12. Almekinders LC, Tao MA, Zarzour R. Playing hurt: hand and wrist injuries and protected return to sport. Sports Med Arthrosc Rev 2014;22(1):66–70.

13. Grewal R, King G. Percutaneous screw fixation led to faster recovery and return to work than immobilization for fractures of the waist of the scaphoid. J Bone Joint Surg Am 2008;90:1793.

14. Goffin JS, Liao Q, Robertson GA. Return to sport following scaphoid fractures: a systematic review and meta-analysis. World J Orthop 2019;10(2):101–14.

15. De Vos J, Vandenberghe D. Acute percutaneous scaphoid fixation using a non-cannulated Herbert screw. Chir Main 2003;22(2):78–83.

16. Ibrahim T, Qureshi A, Sutton AJ, et al. Surgical versus nonsurgical treatment of acute minimally displaced and undisplaced scaphoid waist fractures: pairwise and network meta-analyses of randomized controlled trials. J Hand Surg Am 2011; 36(11):1759–68.

17. Bushnell MD, McWilliams AD, Messer TM. Complications in dorsal percutaneous cannulated screw fixation of nondisplaced scaphoid waist fractures. J Hand Surg Am 2007;32(6):827–33.

18. Kang KB, Kim HJ, Park JH, et al. Comparison of dorsal and volar percutaneous approaches in acute scaphoid fractures: a meta-analysis. PLoS One 2016;11(9):e0162779.

19. Chan KW, McAdams TR. Central screw placement in percutaneous screw scaphoid fixation: a cadaveric comparison of proximal and distal techniques. J Hand Surg Am 2004;29(1):74–9.

20. McCallister WV, Knight J, Kaliappan R, et al. Central placement of the screw in simulated fractures of the scaphoid waist: a biomechanical study. J Bone Joint Surg Am 2003;85-A(1):72–7.

21. Meermans G, Van Glabbeek F, Braem MJ, et al. Comparison of two percutaneous volar approaches for screw fixation of scaphoid waist fractures: radiographic and biomechanical study of an osteotomy-simulated model. J Bone Joint Surg Am 2014; 96(16):1369–76.

22. Dodds SD, Rush AJ 3rd, Staggers JR. A mini-open, dorsal approach for scaphoid fracture fixation with a ligament sparing arthrotomy. Tech Hand Up Extrem Surg 2020;24(1):32–6.

23. Verstreken F, Meermans G. Transtrapezial approach for fixation of acute scaphoid fractures: rationale, surgical techniques, and results: AAOS exhibit selection. J Bone Joint Surg Am 2015; 97(10):850–8.

24. [Geissler WB, Hammit MD. Arthroscopic aided fixation of scaphoid fractures. Hand Clin 2001;17(4): 575–88.

25. Slutsky DJ. Arthroscopically assisted percutaneous scaphoid screw insertion. In: Slutsky DJ, Slade J, editors. The scaphoid. 1st edition. New York: Thieme; 2011. p. 122–30.

26. Della Rosa N, Lancelotti E, Pilla F, et al. Scaphoid fractures with scapholunate ligamebt involvement: instability or ligamentous laxity? Role of arthroscopy and pinning. Musculoskelet Surg 2019;103:23–6.

27. Slade JF 3rd, Gutow AP, Geissler WB. Percutaneous internal fixation of scaphoid fractures via an arthroscopically assisted dorsal approach. J Bone Joint Surg Am 2002;84- A(Suppl):21–36.

28. Alshryda S, Shah A, Odak S, et al. Acute fractures of the scaphoid bone: systematic review and meta-analysis. Surgeon 2012;10:218–29.

29. Buijze GA, Doornberg JN, Ham JS, et al. Surgical compared with conservative treatment for acute nondisplaced or minimally displaced scaphoid fractures: a systematic review and meta-analysis of randomized controlled trials. J Bone Joint Surg Am 2010;92:1534–44.

30. Garcia RM, Ruch DS. Management of scaphoid fractures in the athlete: open and percutaneous fixation. Sports Med Arthrosc Rev 2014;22(1):22–8.

31. Brekke AC, Snoddy MC, Lee DH, et al. Biomechanical strength of the scaphoid partial union. J Wrist Surg 2018;7(5):399–403.

32. Riester JN, Baker BE, Mosher JF, et al. A review of scaphoid fracture healing in competitive athletes. Am J Sports Med 1985;13(3):159–61.

Shoulder and Elbow

Current Trends and Impact of Early Sports Specialization in the Throwing Athlete

Forrest L. Anderson, MD[a], Michael L. Knudsen, MD[b],
Christopher S. Ahmad, MD[a], Charles A. Popkin, MD[a,*]

KEYWORDS

• Early sports specialization • Throwing athlete • Youth sports injury

---

KEY POINTS

• There is no strong evidence that early sports specialization is a requirement to achieve elite athletic status in throwing sports.
• Early sports specialization is associated with increased injury risk in general, but especially in throwing athletes.
• Athletes who have specialized early have increased rates of burnout and lower rates of lifelong sports participation.
• Parents and coaches strongly influence the developing athlete's choice to specialize early, often to the athlete's detriment.
• Athletes allowed to diversify their sports participation have been shown to benefit both physically and psychologically and progress more frequently to elite levels of play.

INTRODUCTION/BACKGROUND

Organized youth athletics in the United States has increased greatly in both participation and level of competition over the past several decades.[1–4] This shift has morphed what was once a formative hobby for many children with sandlot baseball and free play into a nationwide collection of pre-pubescent semiprofessional sports leagues.[5–7] As parents and coaches strive for an advantage in this evolving and competitive landscape, early sports specialization (ESS) has become an increasingly common trend.[8] Paradoxically, ESS has been shown to be associated with increased rates of burnout, overuse injuries, increased psychological stress, and discontinuation of sport.[9]

HISTORY

The historic basis for the shift to ESS can be traced back to the athletic success of the Olympic programs of formerly communist Eastern European counties.[10] Western media coverage of their successes often emphasized the young age of many of the athletes from those countries, which created the perception that early specialization was both beneficial and required. Many of the coaches who emigrated to the West from these countries also brought and instituted year-round, specialized training programs with them.[11] Many of the sports in which those countries and coaches were most successful, however, are so called "early-entry sports," such as gymnastics, diving,

---

[a] Department of Orthopedic Surgery, Columbia University Medical Center, 622 West 168th Street PH-11, New York, NY 10032, USA; [b] Department of Orthopedic Surgery, University of Minnesota, 2450 Riverside Avenue South, Suite R200, Minneapolis, MN 55454, USA
* Corresponding author.
E-mail address: cp2654@cumc.columbia.edu

Orthop Clin N Am 51 (2020) 517–525
https://doi.org/10.1016/j.ocl.2020.06.006
0030-5898/20/© 2020 Elsevier Inc. All rights reserved.

dance, and figure skating, where athletes often peak at an earlier age than in most other sports,[12] and their successes were much more broadly applied.

The popular perception that 10,000 hours of deliberate practice is required to achieve mastery in skill-based disciplines such as music or chess[13] has also been applied to sports and used as a rationalization for early specialization.[14] Although research has shown that the "10,000 hour rule" does not necessarily apply to sports,[15] it has likely led to parents pressuring their children to specialize in one sport earlier to get a head start on that timeframe.

Parents have been shown to be a driving factor leading to ESS.[16] Whether it be for the possibility of future financial gains through the pursuit of college scholarships and professional contracts,[10] or the just for the general perceived success of raising an expert level athlete.

DEFINITIONS

- Broadly, ESS is defined as "intense, year-round training in a single sport at the exclusion of other sports."[17]

Other definitions offer more specific conditions, including the following criteria published in a recent consensus statement by The American Orthopedic Society for Sports Medicine[18]:

1. Participation in intensive training and/or competition in organized sport for more than 8 months per year, or approximately year-round.
2. Participation in one sport to the exclusion of participation in other sport or limited free play.
3. Involving prepubertal children, seventh grade, and/or younger than age 12 years.

A sports specialization scale has also been published,[19] offering 1 point for answering "yes" to each of the following questions:

1. Does the athlete participate in the sport more than 8 months per year?
2. Has the athlete quit other sports to focus on one primary sport?
3. Is your primary sport more important than other sports?

A score of 2 indicates "moderate specialization," while a score of 3 indicates "high specialization." Athletes meeting the definition of "high specialization" were shown to be at a higher risk of serious overuse injury compared with lower-scoring athletes (Table 1).

Table 1
Sports specialization score baseball

3 Questions Asked:	Scoring	Total Score = Level of Specialization
Does the athlete participate in the sport >8 mo?	1 point for yes, 0 for no	0–1 total score = Low Specialization
Has the athlete quit other sports to focus on baseball?	1 point for yes, 0 for no	2 Moderate Specialization
Is baseball more important than other sports?	1 point for yes, 0 for no	3 High Specialization

Adapted with permission from Jayanthi NA, LaBella CR, Fischer D, Pasulka J, Dugas LR: Sports-specialized intensive training and the risk of injury in young athletes: A clinical case-control study. Am J Sports Med 2015;43:794-801.

DISCUSSION
General Problems with Early Sports Specialization

Evidence has shown that ESS increases the risk for both negative physical and psychological development of the youth athlete while actually decreasing the likelihood of progressing to an elite level and increasing rates of dropout.

Injury

Ruedl and colleagues[20] examined 1206 7-year-olds to 18-year-olds over 3 years and showed that focusing on a single main sport was an independent risk factor for injury after controlling for age and time participating in sports activity with an odds ratio of 1.48. Hall and colleagues[21] concluded that ESS was associated with a 1.5 times increased risk of anterior knee pain after following a cohort of 546 adolescent female athletes. Post and colleagues[22] demonstrated that athletes scoring high on the sport specialization scale were more likely to report any injury (odds ratio [OR] 1.59) or overuse injury (OR 1.45) than youth athletes in the low specialization group in a series of more than 2000 athletes aged 12 to 18.

In a recent prospective MRI study looking for shoulder abnormalities in young baseball players, increased risk was found in those who played baseball year-round and/or made the All-Star Team, as opposed to the hypothesized factors of pitch counts and position played.[23]

Burnout
Athlete burnout is a psychological syndrome that is manifested by a reduced sense of accomplishment, emotional/physical exhaustion, and devaluation of participation in sport.[24] There is growing evidence that ESS may be associated with increased burnout.[25–28]

Specialized athletes are at risk of developing burnout because of increased demands to play their particular sport, increased critical performance evaluations, and high rates of overtraining.[29–31] A study of 376 adolescent athletes across 19 different sports found that 29% had experienced an episode of nonfunctional overreaching or overtraining in their past; such episodes were defined as a significant decrement in performance that persisted for periods of time longer than 2 weeks in the setting of continued training.[32] A burnt-out athlete is unlikely to maintain the motivation or intrinsic drive that has been shown to be essential for achievement and continued participation in sport.[12,33]

Developmental Growth
Multiple studies have sought to elucidate the social and psychological risks of ESS. It is thought that it may limit opportunities for behavioral development, lead to social isolation, and limit opportunities for interpersonal growth because of decreased exposure to peers outside of their given sport.[12,34,35]

Withdrawal from Sport
Padaki and colleagues[36] examined a group of young, specialized athletes and found that 47% of the athletes considered quitting their sport

within the last season. The mean age of sport specialization for study participants was 8.1 years. ESS generally leads to increased training intensity and volume, which has been associated with higher rates of withdrawal from sport in the immature athlete.[32] Excessive training volume or intensity can also curtail enjoyment and prevent long-term sport participation.[27]

Decreased Progression to an Elite Level
Multiple studies comparing elite to near-elite athletes have consistently shown that the elite athletes specialized later than near-elite athletes.[31,37–39] In addition, it has been shown in a study of National Basketball Association first-round draft picks, that those who remained multisport athletes in high school had longer careers and were more likely to avoid major injury than their peers who specialized in basketball early.[1] A recent review of ESS found no clear association between specializing early and elite achievement in numerous sports.[5] In baseball, a recent study compared Major League Baseball (MLB) players who were multisport athletes in high school with those who only played baseball and found that the multisport athletes played in more MLB games and experienced lower injury rates of both upper and lower extremity injuries.[40] Another study looking at ESS and professional baseball found that players who specialized before high school had a significantly higher rate of self-reported serious injury than those players who specialized later.[41]

Alternatives to Early Sports Specialization
The data supporting early diversification in sports is strong. By providing the developing athlete with exposures to many unique

Table 2
MLB.com pitch smart guidelines for the youth and adolescent thrower

Age	Daily Max (Pitches in a Game)	0 Days Rest	1 Days Rest	2 Days Rest	3 Days Rest	4 Days Rest	5 Days Rest
7–8	50	1–20	21–35	36–50	N/A	N/A	N/A
9–10	75	1–20	21–35	36–50	51–65	66+	N/A
11–12	85	1–20	21–35	36–50	51–65	66+	N/A
13–14	95	1–20	21–35	36–50	51–65	66+	N/A
15–16	95	1–30	31–45	46–60	61–75	76+	N/A
17–18	105	1–30	31–45	46–60	61–80	81+	N/A

psychosocial, physical, and cognitive situations,[35] diversification encourages the young athlete to transfer these physical and mental skills from one sport to another.[30,31,42] Cross-training is broadly supported in adult athletes and has been show to improve performance in the developing athlete as well. Fransen and colleagues[43] compared 735 boys, aged 6 to 12 years old, who participated in either a single sport or multiple sports. In the oldest multisport subgroup (10–12-year-olds), significant positive effects in strength and coordination were observed. Baker and Côte[44] also found that

athletes exposed to multiple sports from an early age found more enjoyment in sport and dropped out less frequently than ESS athletes. Enjoyment of the sport is a robust predictor of long-term participation and eventual achievement.[17,44]

Evidence for Late Specialization

With the exception of the early peak performance sports (gymnastics, diving, dance, and figure skating),[6] evidence suggests that ESS is not a requirement for athletic success.[12,31,45,46] Multiple investigations have shown that athletes

---

THE YOUTH THROWING SCORE (YTS)

Name: _____   Email: _____

Age: _____   City, State, Zip: _____ , _____ , _____

Date of Birth: _____ / _____ / _____   Today's Date: _____ / _____ / _____

PART 1

Please answer EACH of the following questions.

1. What is your main sport?   ☐ Baseball   ☐ Tennis   ☐ Other _____

2. What position do you play most often?

    ☐ Pitcher   ☐ Catcher   ☐ 1B   ☐ 2B   ☐ SS   ☐ 3B   ☐ Outfield

3. What other positions do you play?

    ☐ Pitcher   ☐ Catcher   ☐ 1B   ☐ 2B   ☐ SS   ☐ 3B   ☐ Outfield

4. Have you ever had an injury to your throwing arm?   ☐ Yes   ☐ No

    a. If so, what type of injury did you have? _____

    _____

    b. What date (approximately) did this injury occur? _____

5. Have you ever had surgery on your throwing arm?   ☐ Yes   ☐ No

    a. If YES, what type of surgery did you have? _____

    _____

    b. If YES, what date (approximately) did this injury occur? _____

6. What type of league(s) do you play in?

    ☐ School league   ☐ Out-of-School (club) League   ☐ Both Types of leagues

7. Check the box that best describes the pain or discomfort level you felt the last time you played your sport:

    ☐ Playing **without** any arm pain or discomfort

    ☐ Playing **with** arm pain or discomfort

    ☐ **Not** playing due to arm pain or discomfort

Fig. 1. A worksheet used to determine an athlete's Youth Throwing Score. (*Courtesy of* Columbia University Orthopedics.)

PART 2

Please answer EACH of the following questions 14 questions.
*Mark **only one** box for each question*

1. Does your arm hurt when you throw?

☐ Never   ☐ Rarely   ☐ Sometimes   ☐ Often   ☐ Always

2. Does your arm hurt the day after your throw?

☐ Never   ☐ Rarely   ☐ Sometimes   ☐ Often   ☐ Always

3. Does your arm get tired during a game or practice?

☐ Never   ☐ Rarely   ☐ Sometimes   ☐ Often   ☐ Always

4. Does arm pain decrease your throwing accuracy?

☐ Never   ☐ Rarely   ☐ Sometimes   ☐ Often   ☐ Always

5. Does arm pain limit how hard you can throw?

☐ Never   ☐ Rarely   ☐ Sometimes   ☐ Often   ☐ Always

6. Does arm pain or weakness limit the number of <u>innings</u> you can play?

☐ Never   ☐ Rarely   ☐ Sometimes   ☐ Often   ☐ Always

7. Does arm pain or weakness limit the number of <u>games</u> you can play?

☐ Never   ☐ Rarely   ☐ Sometimes   ☐ Often   ☐ Always

8. Does arm pain prevent you from playing on multiple teams or leagues?

☐ Never   ☐ Rarely   ☐ Sometimes   ☐ Often   ☐ Always

9. Does arm pain make it hard to play your favorite position?

☐ Never   ☐ Rarely   ☐ Sometimes   ☐ Often   ☐ Always

10. Has arm pain or weakness forced you to change your throwing motion?

☐ Never   ☐ Rarely   ☐ Sometimes   ☐ Often   ☐ Always

Fig. 1. (continued.)

who progress to the elite levels of their sport do not specialize their training until late adolescence.[31,39]

An athlete's own intrinsic drive has also been shown to be fundamental to achieving elite status.[5] A study conducted on 16-year-old pre-elite soccer players demonstrated that the main difference between the players who eventually went on to play professionally and those who failed was that the future professionals sought out and accumulated more hours of unstructured soccer during their free time.[47]

Specifics to the Throwing Athlete

Many of the specific risks of ESS in the throwing athlete pertain to injury prevalence and prevention. ESS puts athletes at higher risk for overuse injury, and baseball players, chiefly pitchers, are at a uniquely high risk for these injuries.[19,48–50] With more than 100,000 baseball players aged 18 and younger reporting to emergency rooms annually in the United States,[51] some consider this issue to have reached epidemic porportions.[52] Adolescent pitchers are at a much higher risk (4 to 36 times) of sustaining an injury due to overuse or fatigue than their peers, and those who pitched more than 8 months per year have also been shown to undergo more shoulder and elbow surgeries.[53] Pitchers who throw more than 75 pitches in a game have increased rates of reported shoulder pain.[10] Elbow injuries in pitchers are correlated

PART 2   *continued*

11. Does arm <u>pain</u> cause you to have less fun while playing?

☐ Never   ☐ Rarely   ☐ Sometimes   ☐ Often   ☐ Always

12. Does arm <u>weakness</u> cause you to have less fun while playing?

☐ Never   ☐ Rarely   ☐ Sometimes   ☐ Often   ☐ Always

13. Does arm <u>pain</u> hold you back from being a better player?

☐ Never   ☐ Rarely   ☐ Sometimes   ☐ Often   ☐ Always

14. Does arm <u>weakness</u> hold you back from being a better player?

☐ Never   ☐ Rarely   ☐ Sometimes   ☐ Often   ☐ Always

Fig. 1. (continued.)

with pitching volume, pitching fatigue, and increased elbow torque related to poor mechanics,[54] and although the overall injury rate in youth baseball is decreasing, the rate of elbow injuries in adolescents is actually increasing.[9] In all age groups, overuse has been found to be the main cause of ulnar collateral ligament injury.[55] In response to these data, leadership organizations in youth baseball instituted recommended pitch count limitations in 2001, with specific recommendations stratified to the age of the players.[53,56] Despite these recommendations, in 2012 Ahmad and colleagues[57] reported that 31% of baseball coaches, 28% of players, and 25% of parents do not believe that pitch counts are a risk factor for elbow injury. In baseball-heavy South Carolina, a recent study highlighted that only 58% of parents were aware of pitch count guidelines.[58] Despite the institution of these recommended pitch counts[59] (Table 2) and the direct relationship between overuse and ulnar collateral ligament injury, the rate of reported ulnar collateral ligament injuries in youth baseball pitchers continues to rise exponentially.[60] As recently as 2014, it seems a significant contributor to this epidemic may simply be a lack of consistent pitch count enforcement. A study of 754 pitchers from 9 to 18 years of age found that nearly half had no pitch counts restrictions in place, and 13% were pitching for more than 8 months per year.[61] In addition, Fazarale and colleagues[62] surveyed 228 coaches with regard to pitch count rules and they incorrectly answered 57% of questions.

In the hopes of creating a standardized measuring tool to help further understand the injury burden related to ESS and in youth baseball in general, Ahmad and colleagues[60] produced and validated the "Youth Throwing Score" (YTS). Using this tool, the investigators reported that 45.3% of the 223 baseball players aged 10 to 18 they studied described an injury to their throwing arm (**Fig. 1**). The YTS is easy to administer and can identify young throwers pitching with pain. The mean score of players throwing without pain was 60, whereas the mean score of those throwing with pain was 42.[60] The use of such an assessment tool can both further future research endeavors, and hope to assist health care providers in decreasing the rates of these injuries. Furthermore, another research concept that has gained more attention is the concept of Acute to Chronic Workload Ratio (ACWR), or the ratio of acute workload in 1 week compared with the previous 4 weeks.[63] It has been postulated that an acute rise in the ACWR can be correlated with increased injury risk.[64] The concept of ACWR spikes in the young throwing athlete warrants future study, as it may be an essential link to predicting fatigue and lowering the rates of injury in this at-risk population.[64,65]

SUMMARY

- ESS remains a passionate topic. Many parents and coaches continue to advocate the practice of ESS, despite the data showing that it is not required for development of the young, aspiring throwing athlete.
- Although orthopedic surgeons and sports medicine physicians have traditionally only been concerned with injury treatment and prevention, more and more patients and their families are

turning to their health care providers for guidance to help achieve peak performance.

- It is important to remember that although many coaches and parents encouraging ESS may not be acting in their young athlete's best interest, they are well intentioned; they want their child to become as good at their given sport as possible. Their goals are actually aligned with providers. However, they may not fully understand the evidence behind sport specialization. Keeping this in mind, it is crucial to develop a therapeutic alliance with parents and coaches. The data seem to show that early diversification of sport should be encouraged, whereas sport specialization should be delayed until at least late adolescence.
- The most current data show that delaying sport specialization decreases risk of injury, burnout, and discontinuation of sport while increasing the psychological and physical development of the athlete and increasing their chances of progressing to elite status.

CLINICS CARE POINTS

- There is no strong evidence that early sports specialization is a requirement to achieve elite athletic status in throwing sports.
- Early sports specialization is associated with increased injury risk in general, but especially in the throwing athlete.
- Athletes who have specialized early have increased rates of burnout and lower rates of lifelong sports participation.
- Parents and coaches strongly influence the developing athlete's choice to specialize early, often to the athlete's detriment.
- Athletes allowed to diversify their sports participation have been shown to benefit both physically and psychologically and progress more frequently to elite levels of play.
- Encourage free play and late specialization in baseball until the high school level.

DISCLOSURE

Dr F.L. Anderson has nothing to disclose. Dr M.L. Knudsen is a team physician for the Minnesota Twins. Dr C.S. Ahmad or immediate family member is a consultant for, receives educational support from, is a paid speaker/presenter for, and receives research support from Arthrex; receives research support from Major League Baseball and Stryker; receives royalties from Arthrex and Lead Player; has received hospitality payments from Arthrex and DePuy Synthes; and has stock/stock options in At Peak. He is the head team physician for the New York Yankees. Dr C.A Popkin or an immediate family member has received educational support from Arthrex and has received hospitality payments from Smith & Nephew, Arthrex, and Gotham Surgical Solutions and Devices.

REFERENCES

1. Rugg C, Kadoor A, Feeley BT, et al. The effects of playing multiple high school sports on national basketball association players' propensity for injury and athletic performance. Am J Sports Med 2018; 46(2):402–8.

2. Sheu Y, Chen LH, Hedegaard H. Sports-and recreation-related injury episodes in the United States, 2011–2014. Natl Health Stat Rep 2016; 2016(99):1–12.

3. Feeley BT, Agel J, Laprade RF. When is it too early for single sport specialization? Am J Sports Med 2016;44(1):234–41.

4. Zhang AL, Sing DC, Rugg CM, et al. The rise of concussions in the adolescent population. Orthop J Sport Med 2016;4(8). https://doi.org/10.1177/2325967116662458.

5. Popkin CA, Bayomy AF, Ahmad CS. Early sport specialization. J Am Acad Orthop Surg 2019. https://doi.org/10.5435/JAAOS-D-18-00187.

6. Difiori JP, Benjamin HJ, Brenner JS, et al. Overuse injuries and burnout in youth sports: a position statement from the American Medical Society for Sports Medicine. Br J Sports Med 2014;48(4):287–8.

7. Gould D. Editorial: the professionalization of youth sports: it's time to act! Clin J Sport Med 2009;19(2): 81–2.

8. Fabricant PD, Lakomkin N, Sugimoto D, et al. Youth sports specialization and musculoskeletal injury: a systematic review of the literature. Phys Sportsmed 2016;44(3):257–62.

9. Trofa DP, Obana KK, Swindell HW, et al. Increasing burden of youth baseball elbow injuries in US emergency departments. Orthop J Sport Med 2019;7(5):1–6.

10. Malina RM. Early sport specialization: roots, effectiveness, risks. Curr Sports Med Rep 2010;9(6):364–71.

11. Myer GD, Jayanthi N, DiFiori JP, et al. Sports specialization, Part II: alternative solutions to early sport specialization in youth athletes. Sports Health 2016;8(1):65–73.

12. Myer GD, Jayanthi N, Difiori JP, et al. Sport specialization, Part I: does early sports specialization increase negative outcomes and reduce the opportunity for success in young athletes? Sports Health 2015;7(5):437–42.

13. Ericsson KA, Krampe RT, Tesch-Römer C. The role of deliberate practice in the acquisition of expert performance. Psychol Rev 1993. https://doi.org/10.1037/0033-295x.100.3.363.

14. Starkes JL, Ericsson KA. Expert performance in sport: advances in research on sport expertise. Champlain (IL): Human Kinetics; 2003.

15. Fraser-Thomas J, Côté J. Youth sports: implementing findings and moving forward with research. Athl Insight 2006;8(3):12–27.

16. Padaki AS, Popkin CA, Hodgins JL, et al. Factors that drive youth specialization. Sports Health 2017;9(6):532–6.

17. Jayanthi N, Pinkham C, Dugas L, et al. Sports specialization in young athletes: evidence-based recommendations. Sports Health 2013;5(3):251–7.

18. LaPrade RF, Agel J, Baker J, et al. AOSSM early sport specialization consensus statement. Orthop J Sport Med 2016. https://doi.org/10.1177/2325967116644241.

19. Jayanthi NA, Labella CR, Fischer D, et al. Sports-specialized intensive training and the risk of injury in young athletes: a clinical case-control study. Am J Sports Med 2015;43(4):794–801.

20. Ruedl G, Schobersberger W, Pocecco E, et al. Sport injuries and illnesses during the first Winter Youth Olympic Games 2012 in Innsbruck, Austria. Br J Sports Med 2012. https://doi.org/10.1136/bjsports-2012-091534.

21. Hall R, Foss KB, Hewett TE, et al. Sport specialization's association with an increased risk of developing anterior knee pain in adolescent female athletes. J Sport Rehabil 2015. https://doi.org/10.1123/jsr.2013-0101.

22. Post EG, Trigsted SM, Riekena JW, et al. The Association of Sport Specialization and Training volume with injury history in youth athletes. Am J Sports Med 2017. https://doi.org/10.1177/0363546517690848.

23. Holt JB, Stearns PH, Bastrom TP, et al. The curse of the all-star team: a single-season prospective shoulder MRI study of Little League baseball players. J Pediatr Orthop 2019. https://doi.org/10.1097/BPO.0000000000001391.

24. Raedeke TD, Smith AL. Development and preliminary validation of an athlete burnout measure. J Sport Exerc Psychol 2001. https://doi.org/10.1123/jsep.23.4.281.

25. Joel S. Brenner Sports specialization and intensive training in young athlete. Pediatrics 2016;138(3):e20162148-e20162148.

26. Goodger K, Gorely T, Lavallee D, et al. Burnout in sport: a systematic review. The Sport Psychologist 2007;21:127-51.

27. Mostafavifar AM, Best TM, Myer GD. Early sport specialisation, does it lead to long-term problems? Br J Sports Med 2013. https://doi.org/10.1136/bjsports-2012-092005.

28. Fraser-Thomas J, Cote J, Deakin J. Examining adolescent sport dropout and prolonged engagement from a developmental perspective. J Appl Sport Psychol 2008. https://doi.org/10.1080/10413200802163549.

29. Gould D, Tuffey S, Udry E, et al. Burnout in competitive junior tennis players: I. A quantitative psychological assessment. Sport Psychol 1996. https://doi.org/10.1123/tsp.10.4.322.

30. Baker J, Côté J, Abernethy B. Sport-specific practice and the development of expert decision-making in team ball sports. J Appl Sport Psychol 2003. https://doi.org/10.1080/10413200305400.

31. Moesch K, Elbe AM, Hauge MLT, et al. Late specialization: the key to success in centimeters, grams, or seconds (cgs) sports. Scand J Med Sci Sports 2011. https://doi.org/10.1111/j.1600-0838.2010.01280.x.

32. Matos AF, Winsley RJ, Williams CA. Prevalence of nonfunctional overreaching/overtraining in young English athletes. Med Sci Sports Exerc 2011;43(7):1287–94.

33. Cô té J, Baker J, Abernethy B. Practice and play in the development of sport expertise. In: Tenenbaum G, Eklund RC, editors. Handbook of sport psychology. 3rd edition; Hoboken, NJ; John WIley and Sons: 2012;8:184-202. https://doi.org/10.1002/9781118270011.ch8.

34. Patrick H, Ryan AM, Alfeld-Liro C, et al. Adolescents' commitment to developing talent: The role of peers in continuing motivation for sports and the arts. J Youth Adolesc 1999. https://doi.org/10.1023/A:1021643718575.

35. Côté J, Lidor R, Hackfort D. ISSP position stand: to sample or to specialize? Seven postulates about youth sport activities that lead to continued participation and elite performance. Int J Sport Exerc Psychol 2009. https://doi.org/10.1080/1612197X.2009.9671889.

36. Padaki AS, Ahmad CS, Hodgins JL, et al. Quantifying parental influence on youth athlete specialization: a survey of athletes' parents. Orthop J Sport Med 2017;5(9):1–7.

37. Carlson R. The socialization of elite tennis players in Sweden: an analysis of the players' backgrounds and development. Sociol Sport J 2016. https://doi.org/10.1123/ssj.5.3.241.

38. Lidor R, Lavyan NZ. A retrospective picture of early sport experiences among elite and near-elite Israeli athletes: developmental and psychological perspectives. Int J Sport Psychol 2002;33:269–89.

39. Güllich A, Emrich E. Evaluation of the support of young athletes in the elite sports system. Eur J

Sport Soc 2006. https://doi.org/10.1080/16138171.2006.11687783.

40. Confino J, Irvine JN, O'Connor M, et al. Early sports specialization is associated with upper extremity injuries in throwers and fewer games played in Major League Baseball. Orthop J Sport Med 2019. https://doi.org/10.1177/2325967119861101.

41. Wilhelm A, Choi C, Deitch J. Early sport specialization: effectiveness and risk of injury in professional baseball players. Orthop J Sport Med 2017. https://doi.org/10.1177/2325967117728922.

42. Williams AM, Ford PR. Expertise and expert performance in sport. Int Rev Sport Exerc Psychol 2008. https://doi.org/10.1080/17509840701836867.

43. Fransen J, Pion J, Vandendriessche J, et al. Differences in physical fitness and gross motor coordination in boys aged 6-12 years specializing in one versus sampling more than one sport. J Sports Sci 2012. https://doi.org/10.1080/02640414.2011.642808.

44. Baker J, Cote J. Shifting training requirements during athlete development: the relationship among deliberate practice, deliberate play and other sport involvement in the acquisition of sport expertise. In: Hackfort D, Tenenbaum G, editors. Essential processes for attaining peak performance. Oxford: Meyer and Meyer Sport; 2006;1(5). p. 92-109.

45. Swindell HW, Marcille ML, Trofa DP, et al. An analysis of sports specialization in NCAA division I collegiate athletics. Orthop J Sport Med 2019. https://doi.org/10.1177/2325967118821179.

46. Buckley PS, Bishop M, Kane P, et al. Early single-sport specialization a survey of 3090 high school, collegiate, and professional athletes. Orthop J Sport Med 2017. https://doi.org/10.1177/2325967117703944.

47. Ford PR, Ward P, Hodges NJ, et al. The role of deliberate practice and play in career progression in sport: the early engagement hypothesis. High Abil Stud 2009. https://doi.org/10.1080/13598130902860721.

48. Brenner JS, LaBella CR, Brooks MA, et al. Sports specialization and intensive training in young athletes. Pediatrics 2016. https://doi.org/10.1542/peds.2016-2148.

49. Lyman S, Fleisig GS, Andrews JR, et al. Effect of pitch type, pitch count, and pitching mechanics on risk of elbow and shoulder pain in youth baseball pitchers. Am J Sports Med 2002. https://doi.org/10.1177/03635465020300040201.

50. Makhni EC, Morrow ZS, Luchetti TJ, et al. Arm pain in youth baseball players: a survey of healthy players. Am J Sports Med 2015. https://doi.org/10.1177/0363546514555506.

51. Lawson BR, Comstock RD, Smith GA. Baseball-related injuries to children treated in hospital emergency departments in the United States, 1994-

2006. Pediatrics 2009. https://doi.org/10.1542/peds.2007-3796.

52. Fleisig GS, Andrews JR, Cutter GR, et al. Risk of serious injury for young baseball pitchers: a 10-year prospective study. Am J Sports Med 2011. https://doi.org/10.1177/0363546510384224.

53. Olsen SJ, Fleisig GS, Dun S, et al. Risk factors for shoulder and elbow injuries in adolescent baseball pitchers. Am J Sports Med 2006. https://doi.org/10.1177/0363546505284188.

54. Fleisig GS, Weber A, Hassell N, et al. Prevention of elbow injuries in youth baseball pitchers. Curr Sports Med Rep 2009. https://doi.org/10.1249/JSR.0b013e3181b7ee5f.

55. Bruce JR, Andrews JR. Ulnar collateral ligament injuries in the throwing athlete. J Am Acad Orthop Surg 2014. https://doi.org/10.5435/JAAOS-22-05-315.

56. Dun S, Fleisig GS, Loftice J, et al. The relationship between age and baseball pitching kinematics in professional baseball pitchers. J Biomech 2007. https://doi.org/10.1016/j.jbiomech.2006.01.008.

57. Ahmad CS, Jeffrey Grantham W, Michael Greiwe R. Public perceptions of Tommy John surgery. Phys Sportsmed 2012. https://doi.org/10.3810/psm.2012.05.1966.

58. Eichinger JK, Goodloe JB, Lin JJ, et al. Pitch count adherence and injury assessment of youth baseball in South Carolina. J Orthop 2020. https://doi.org/10.1016/j.jor.2020.01.049.

59. Feeley BT, Schisel J, Agel J. Pitch counts in youth baseball and softball: a historical review. Clin J Sport Med 2018. https://doi.org/10.1097/JSM.0000000000000446.

60. Ahmad CS, Padaki AS, Noticewala MS, et al. The youth throwing score. Am J Sports Med 2017; 45(2):317–24.

61. Yang J, Mann BJ, Guettler JH, et al. Risk-prone pitching activities and injuries in youth baseball: Findings from a national sample. Am J Sports Med 2014. https://doi.org/10.1177/0363546514524699.

62. Fazarale JJ, Magnussen RA, Pedroza AD, et al. Knowledge of and compliance with pitch count recommendations: A survey of youth baseball coaches. Sports Health 2012. https://doi.org/10.1177/1941738111435632.

63. Hulin BT, Gabbett TJ, Blanch P, et al. Spikes in acute workload are associated with increased injury risk in elite cricket fast bowlers. Br J Sports Med 2014. https://doi.org/10.1136/bjsports-2013-092524.

64. Zaremski JL, Zeppieri G, Tripp BL. Sport specialization and overuse injuries in adolescent throwing athletes: A narrative review. J Athl Train 2019. https://doi.org/10.4085/1062-6050-333-18.

65. Black GM, Gabbett TJ, Cole MH, et al. Monitoring workload in throwing-dominant sports: a systematic review. Sports Med 2016. https://doi.org/10.1007/s40279-016-0529-6.

Pulmonary Comorbidities Are Associated with Increased Major Complication Rates Following Indwelling Interscalene Nerve Catheters for Shoulder Arthroplasty

Ian Power, MD[a], Thomas W. Throckmorton, MD[b],
Richard A. Smith, PhD[b], Frederick M. Azar, MD[b],
Tyler J. Brolin, MD[b],*

KEYWORDS

- Shoulder arthroplasty • Pain management • Indwelling interscalene catheter
- Interscalene nerve block • Complications • Pulmonary comorbidities

---

KEY POINTS

- Indwelling interscalene nerve catheters (ISCs), single-shot interscalene nerve blocks (ISBs), and periarticular injections have all shown to be effective for pain control after total shoulder arthroplasty (TSA).
- Pulmonary comorbidities and ASA physical status class III and IV can significantly increase the rate of major complications following ISC placement.
- Patients with an underlying pulmonary comorbidity or lung disease (chronic obstructive pulmonary disease, asthma, or obstructive sleep apnea) have a 2.2-fold increased risk of having any complication and a 2.4-fold increased risk of having a major pulmonary complication compared to those without pulmonary comorbidities.
- Patients with pulmonary comorbidities may benefit from alternative pain management strategies to avoid complications in the early postoperative period.

INTRODUCTION

One of the greatest advances in the perioperative management of patients undergoing total joint arthroplasty has been the improvement in postoperative pain management strategies. Today, much of the emphasis is on providing effective postoperative pain control while limiting opioid-based pain medications. This has the advantage of avoiding the side effects and dependency issues associated with narcotic pain medications. Commonly seen side effects from predominantly opioid-based pain regimens, such as nausea, vomiting, constipation, respiratory depression, sedation, and delirium, can jeopardize patient safety and increase length of stay after total joint arthroplasty.[1,2]

No funds were received in support of this study. Neither the authors nor their immediate family received any financial payments or other benefits from any commercial entity related to the subject of this article. This study was approved by the University of Tennessee Health Science Center Institutional Review Board: # 16-04580-XP.

[a] Orthopedic Associates P.A., Farmington, NM, USA; [b] Department of Orthopaedic Surgery and Biomedical Engineering, University of Tennessee-Campbell Clinic, Memphis, TN, USA

* Corresponding author. University of Tennessee-Campbell Clinic, 1211 Union Avenue, Suite 510, Memphis, TN 38104.

E-mail address: tbrolin@campbellclinic.com

Also, with the rising rates of opioid abuse, opioid-related fatalities, and economic burden of treating the opioid epidemic, the prescribing patterns of narcotic pain medications have fallen under scrutiny, and health care providers have sought alternative pain management strategies that limit narcotic pain medication use.

Currently, there is no clear consensus on the optimal pain management strategy after shoulder arthroplasty. Multimodal approaches to pain management may include anti-inflammatories, acetaminophen, and pregabalin or gabapentin in combination with an interscalene single-shot nerve block (ISB), indwelling interscalene catheter (ISC), or periarticular injection with liposomal bupivacaine. All 3 strategies have been used with good success at treating perioperative pain[3–5] and limiting side effects while improving patient satisfaction after shoulder arthroplasty.[6,7] Recent investigations comparing interscalene blockade with periarticular injection have focused on the effects of each on early postoperative pain control and narcotic requirements after shoulder arthroplasty.[8,9]

Potential pulmonary complications after phrenic nerve blockade after ISC placement remain a concern. Currently, there is a paucity of literature regarding patient factors as they relate to complications after ISC. A better understanding of which factors place patients at increased risk of complications after ISC will aid surgeons in determining which patients would benefit from alternative pain management strategies. The authors sought to investigate the complication rates with the use of ISCs and determine which patient comorbidities and factors may place patients at increased risk for a complication after shoulder arthroplasty.

MATERIALS AND METHODS

After institutional review board approval, an institutional database review identified 154 patients who had primary shoulder arthroplasty (anatomic total shoulder arthroplasty [TSA] and reverse TSA [RTSA]) and in whom an ISC was used for postoperative pain control between March 2011 and March 2014. All patients were approved for indwelling ISCs by a staff anesthesiologist. The ISC was placed under ultrasound guidance by the anesthesia team, using an 18-gauge needle to infiltrate the brachial plexus trunks, with 20 mL of 0.5% bupivacaine with 1:200,000 epinephrine from a lateral approach. ISCs were kept in place 3 days to 4 days postoperatively unless a complication necessitated removal.

All shoulder arthroplasties were performed by an experienced, fellowship-trained shoulder and elbow surgeon with the patient in the beach chair position under general anesthesia. A standard deltopectoral approach was used and the subscapularis was managed with a tenotomy when present. Standard procedures for both TSA and RTSA included deltoid mobilization and standard releases. After implantation of components, the subscapularis was repaired with transosseous drill holes for TSA and a soft tissue repair when possible for RTSA.

Each patient's medical record was reviewed for pulmonary complications, mechanical catheter-related complications, medical comorbidities, American Society of Anesthesiologists (ASA) class, age, and body mass index (BMI). Major pulmonary complications included death, respiratory distress, pneumonia, decreased oxygen saturation, and shortness of breath. Minor complications included malfunctioning catheters, early discontinuation of the catheter (before postoperative day 3), and hematoma at the catheter site.

Chi-square tests were applied to determine associations with major and minor complications, and analysis of variance regression was used to analyze demographic data. Differences were considered statistically significant for values $P<.05$.

RESULTS
Study Group Demographics
In the cohort of 154 patients, 83 had TSA and 71 had RTSA. Arthroplasty was performed on the right shoulder of 85 patients and on the left shoulder of 69 patients. There were no significant demographic differences between patients who had no complications, a major complication, a minor complication, or both a major and a minor complication.

Complications
The overall complication rate was 22.7% (35 of 154); 25 (16.2%) of these were mechanical complications associated with catheter dysfunction, such as catheter leaking, pump malfunction, or early discontinuation, and were classified as minor. Major pulmonary complications, including 1 death, occurred in 6.5% of patients (10 of 154) (Table 1). The death was related to postoperative pneumonia and cerebrovascular accident. A second death related to cardiac arrest occurred in the cohort and was excluded from analysis, given there was no associated pulmonary complication.

Table 1	
Major and minor complications in 154 patients	
Minor complications (16%)	
Mechanical complications associated with catheter dysfunction Catheter leaking Pump malfunction Early discontinuation of ISC	25
Major complications (12%)	
Pulmonary Decreased oxygen saturation Respiratory distress Pneumonia (1 with CVA, resulting in death)	10
Neurologic Altered mental status Seizures Severe shooting pain in the superficial radial nerve distribution	3
Cardiac Cardiac arrest (resulting in death) Stent placement	2
Hematologic Anemia Deep vein thrombosis	2
Incarcerated catheter requiring surgical removal	1

American Society of Anesthesiologists Physical Status Class and Comorbidities

A majority of patients were ASA class II (68) and III (79), 6 were ASA class IV, and 1 was ASA class I (Table 2). There were 10 major pulmonary complications, all occurring in patients with ASA class III or class IV (11.8%, 10 of 85), compared with no complications in 69 ASA class I or class II patients ($P = .001$). Minor complications also were more common in ASA class III and class IV patients, 23.5% (20 of 85), than in ASA class I and class II, 11.6% (8 of 69; $P = .001$).

Patients who had an underlying pulmonary comorbidity or lung disease (chronic obstructive pulmonary disease, asthma, or obstructive sleep apnea) had a 2.2-fold increased risk of having any complication compared with those without pulmonary comorbidities (40.0% vs 18.3%, respectively) and a 2.4-fold increased risk of having a major pulmonary complication (11.1% vs 4.6%, respectively) ($P = .08$) (Table 3). Patients with asthma had a 3-fold increased risk of major complications (15.8% vs 5.2%) and a 2-fold

increased risk in minor complications (31.6% vs 16.3%, respectively; $P = .039$). There was a trend toward higher BMI in those with major complications compared with those without complications (mean BMI 35.1 vs 31.4, respectively; $P = .066$).

Age, gender, diabetes, heart disease, and hypertension were not related to the risk of any complication.

DISCUSSION

Multimodal analgesia is a well-accepted method for pain management after total joint arthroplasty, and, in an effort to limit opioid-based pain medication, research continues to determine which techniques are most effective.[10] ISCs are a frequent choice for postoperative analgesia after TSA, but multiple reports have documented complications with these devices.[11–15] Problems with the catheter generally are minor complications; however, these can be severe. There are case reports of cervical root avulsion, intrathecal catheter placement, and shearing and separating of the polyurethane sheath over the steel wire of the catheter.[12,13,16,17] Other reported complications include nerve damage, respiratory distress or depression with phrenic nerve blockade, and pneumothorax.[11,14,15]

Despite the volume of reports on complications associated with ISCs and ISBs, there is little information on risk factors associated with these complications. Transient phrenic nerve palsy reportedly occurs in 13% to 100% of blocks, whereas persistent phrenic nerve palsy is rare and may have an association with cervical spinal stenosis.[18] One large retrospective review concluded that BMI greater than 25 kg/m² and ASA class IV increased the risk of failure among all types of regional blocks, including ISBs.[19] The authors found that patients with ASA class III or class IV, a marker of increased medical comorbidities, did have a substantial risk of increased major and minor complications compared with those with ASA class I or class II. Additionally, patients with preexisting asthma were at higher risk for both major and minor complications.

Although the authors did not find statistical significance between BMI and complications, there was a trend toward higher BMI in patients who had a major complication. These were pulmonary in nature, and there is some evidence that obese patients (BMI >29 kg/m²) have greater reductions in forced vital capacity and forced expiratory volume in the first second of

Table 2
Complications according to American Society of Anesthesiologists classification

	American Society of Anesthesiologists Class I/II	American Society of Anesthesiologists Class III/IV
Overall complications	11	32
Major complications	3	15
Minor complications	8	17
No complications	58	53
Total	69	85

ASA: Pearson chi-square, $P = .007$.

Classes I and II, 69 patients: 11/69 (15.9%)—complication, 3/69 (4.3%)—major complication, 8/69 (11.6%)—minor complication, and 58/69 (84.0%)—no complication.

Classes III and IV, 85 patients: 32/85 (37.6%)—complication, 15/85 (17.6%)—major complication, 17/85 (14.45%)—minor complication, and 53/85 (62.35%)—no complication.

expiration after ISB for shoulder surgery compared with normal-weight patients (BMI <25 kg/m^2; $P = .046$ and $P = .02$, respectively). Despite these reductions, there was no change in clinical complications or pulmonary events.[20]

Other investigators have shown extremely low rates of complications with ISCs. A prospective study of 1505 patients with ISCs showed effective analgesia and few serious complications.[21] Less than 1% of patients had respiratory failure. After discharge, 27% of patients noted dyspnea, which generally was mild and well tolerated; 14% had numbness or tingling 1 week after surgery, and that number steadily decreased to 0.7% beyond 12 months. In a small, double-blind randomized controlled trial, patients using continuous ISCs after TSA used significantly less opioids and had better pain scores than those who had a single-shot ISB.[3] There were no complications in the 16 patients, and patients with continuous ISC were able to avoid the use of patient-controlled analgesia pumps because of lower pain scores and limited narcotic usage.

A prospective randomized controlled trial evaluated liposomal bupivacaine for single-shot ISB compared with continuous ISCs.[7] Equivalent outcomes were noted between the 2 groups in the first 24 hours, but the continuous ISC group had a higher complication rate (19.4% vs 5.9%, respectively); all complications were minor and were related to catheter malposition or early displacement. A retrospective review of 697 patients comparing single-shot ISBs to ISCs in shoulder or elbow arthroplasty noted pulmonary complications were the most frequent (84%) of the overall complication rate of 13%.[22] There was no significant difference between ISBs and ISCs in terms of serious complications, although those with an ISC were more likely to have a barrier to discharge and a slightly longer length of stay. A meta-analysis looking at the effectiveness of ISBs and ISCs as well as side-effects and complications noted an 11.0% to 11.7% decrease in respiratory indices with ISCs[23]; however, these were documented in only 2 studies.[24,25] One study noted no respiratory complications,[6] whereas the other had a 50% rate of complications consisting of hypoxemia with oxygen saturation less than 90%.[24] There was no documentation of hypoxemia in the ISB group. The investigators concluded that the clinical importance of these changes was uncertain,

Table 3
Complications in patients with and without pulmonary comorbidities

	With Pulmonary Comorbidities	Without Pulmonary Comorbidities
Overall complications	20 (44.4%)	23 (21.1%)
Major complications	8 (17.8.%)	10 (9.2%)
Minor complications	12 (26.7%)	13 (11.9%)
No complications	25 (55.6%)	86 (78.9%)
Total	45	109

Pearson chi-square, $P = .013$.

and that ISCs provided better analgesia up to 48 hours compared with single-shot ISB.[23,24]

Despite good analgesia from both ISBs and ISCs, the reported complications with ISCs have affected surgeon perception. A survey of the American Shoulder and Elbow Surgeons demonstrated that 76% of surgeons would recommend ISBs to their patients undergoing shoulder surgery. When asked about surgeon preference for the type of anesthesia if they were having shoulder surgery, 59% would have a single-shot ISB, whereas 15% would have an ISC, and 26% would not have either type; persistent neuropathy was the more frequently listed concern.[26]

Compared with periarticular liposomal bupivicaine, ISCs have been shown to have significantly higher complication rates and increased cost, with equivalent pain relief and overall outpatient narcotic usage.[27] In a review of 214 shoulder arthroplasties, major and minor complications were more frequent in the ISC group than in the liposomal bupivacaine group ($P = .045$).[27]

The authors' study has several limitations. First, this was a retrospective review with the inherent biases of a retrospective study. The authors conducted a thorough review of clinical records both in the inpatient and outpatient setting, but it is possible some complications were treated at outlying facilities and not recognized. Although patients with an increased number of pulmonary comorbidities had more complications with ISCs, no direct conclusion can be drawn given the lack of a control group. This is 1 institution's results with ISCs for shoulder arthroplasty and may not reflect the experiences of other surgeons and institutions.

SUMMARY

Postoperative pain management after shoulder arthroplasty is without consensus and largely up to surgeon preference. Among studies of ISCs, complication rates vary dramatically and predominantly are catheter-related complications. Of the major complications, most are pulmonary complications. Patients with underlying pulmonary comorbidities and an ASA class III or class IV have an increased risk of sustaining a major complication after the use of an ISC for shoulder arthroplasty. These patients may benefit from alternative pain management strategies, including periarticular injection or single-shot ISB, to avoid complications in the early postoperative period.

REFERENCES

1. Jin F, Chung F. Multimodal analgesia for postoperative pain control. J Clin Anesth 2001;13:524–39.
2. Watcha MF, White PF. Postoperative nausea and vomiting. Its etiology, treatment, and prevention. Anesthesiology 1992;77:162–84.
3. Kean J, Wigderowitz CA, Coventry DM. Continuous interscalene infusion and single injection using levobupivacaine for analgesia after surgery of the shoulder. A double-blind, randomised controlled trial. J Bone Joint Surg Br 2006;88:1173–7.
4. Singh A, Kelly C, O'Brien T, et al. Ultrasound-guided interscalene block anesthesia for shoulder arthroscopy: a prospective study of 1319 patients. J Bone Joint Surg Am 2012;94:2040–6.
5. Swenson JD, Bay N, Loose E, et al. Outpatient management of continuous peripheral nerve catheters placed using ultrasound guidance: an experience in 620 patients. Anesth Analg 2006;103: 1436–43.
6. Abildgaard JT, Lonergan KT, Tolan SJ, et al. Liposomal bupivacaine versus indwelling interscalene nerve block for postoperative pain control in shoulder arthroplasty: a prospective randomized controlled trial. J Shoulder Elbow Surg 2017;26: 1175–81.
7. Sabesan VJ, Shahriar R, Petersen-Fitts GR, et al. A prospective randomized controlled trial to identify the optimal postoperative pain management in shoulder arthroplasty: liposomal bupivacaine versus continuous interscalene catheter. J Shoulder Elbow Surg 2017;26:1810–7.
8. Namdari S, Nicholson T, Abboud J, et al. Randomized controlled trial of interscalene block compared with injectable liposomal bupivacaine in shoulder arthroplasty. J Bone Joint Surg Am 2017;99:550–6.
9. Okoroha KR, Lynch JR, Keller RA, et al. Liposomal bupivacaine versus interscalene nerve block for pain control after shoulder arthroplasty: a prospective randomized trial. J Shoulder Elbow Surg 2016; 25:1742–8.
10. Amundson AW, Johnson RL, Abdel MP, et al. A three-arm randomized clinical trial comparing continuous femoral plus single-injection sciatic peripheral nerve blocks versus periarticular injection with ropivacaine or liposomal bupivacaine for patients undergoing total knee arthroplasty. Anesthesiology 2017;126:1139–50.
11. Adhikary SD, Amstrong K, Chin KJ. Perineural entrapment of an interscalene stimulating catheter. Anesth Intensive Care 2012;40:527–30.
12. Azzam MG, Kimzey GW, Phillips GH, et al. Shearing of a continuous interscalene catheter with lancinating symptoms after an interscalene block: a case report. JBJS Case Connect 2013;3:e83.

13. Boezaart AP, Tighe P. New trends in regional anesthesia for shoulder surgery: avoiding devastating complications. Int J Shoulder Surg 2010;4:1–7.

14. Bowens C Jr, Briggs ER, Malchow RJ. Brachial plexus entrapment of interscalene nerve catheter after uncomplicated ultrasound-guided placement. Pain Med 2011;12:1117–20.

15. Lenters TR, Davies J, Matsen FA 3rd. The types and severity of complications associated with interscalene brachial plexus block anesthesia: local and national evidence. J Shoulder Elbow Surg 2007;16:37–387.

16. Wiesmann T, Wallot P, Nentwig L, et al. Separation of stimulating catheters for continuous peripheral regional anesthesia during their removal – two case reports and a critical appraisal of the use of steel-coil containing stimulating catheters. Local Reg Anesth 2015;8:15–9.

17. Yanovski B, Gaitini L, Volodarski D, et al. Catastrophic complication of an interscalene catheter for continuous peripheral nerve block analgesia. Anaesthesia 2012;67:1166–9.

18. Pakala SR, Beckman JD, Lyman S, et al. Cervical spine disease is a risk factor for persistent phrenic nerve paresis following interscalene nerve block. Reg Anesth Pain Med 2013;38:239–42.

19. Cotter JT, Nielsen KC, Guller U, et al. Increased body mass index and ASA physical status IV are risk factors for block failure in ambulatory surgery – an analysis of 9,342 blocks. Can J Anaesth 2004; 51:810–6.

20. Melton MS, Monroe HE, Qi W, et al. Effect of interscalene brachial plexus block on the pulmonary function of obese patients: a prospective, observational cohort study. Anesth Analg 2017;125:313–9.

21. Fredrickson MJ, Leightley P, Wong A, et al. An analysis of 1505 consecutive patients receiving continuous interscalane analgesia at home: a multicenter prospective safety study. Anaesthesia 2016; 71:373–3779.

22. Thompson M, Simonds R, Clinger B, et al. Continuous versus single shot brachial plexus block and their relationship to discharge barriers and length of stay. J Shoulder Elbow Surg 2017;26:656–61.

23. Vorobeichik L, Brull R, Bowry R, et al. Should continuous rather than single-injection interscalene block be routinely offered for major shoulder surgery? A meta-analysis of the analgesic and side effects profiles. Br J Anaesth 2018;120:679–92.

24. Borgeat A, Perschak H, Bird P, et al. Patient-controlled interscalene analgesia with ropivacaine 0.2% versus pataient-controlled intravenous analgesia after major shoulder surgery: effects on diaphragmatic and respiratory function. Anesthesiology 2000;92:102–8.

25. Pere P. The effect of continuous interscalene brachial plexus block with 0.125% bupivacaine plus fentanyl on diaphragmatic motility and ventilator function. Reg Anesth 1993;18:93–7.

26. Moore DD, Maerz T, Anderson K. Shoulder surgeons' perceptions of interscalene nerve blocks and a review of complication rates in the literature. Phys Sportsmed 2013;41:77–84.

27. Weller WJ, Azzam MG, Smith RA, et al. Liposomal bupivacaine mixture has similar pain relief and significantly fewer complications at less cost compared to indwelling interscalene catheter in total shoulder arthroplasty. J Arthroplasty 2017;32: 3557–62.

Foot and Ankle

Management of Achilles Tendon Injuries in the Elite Athlete

Karan A. Patel[a], Martin J. O'Malley[b,*]

KEYWORDS

- Achilles rupture • High-level athletes • Elite athletes • Surgical intervention

KEY POINTS

- Achilles tendon ruptures typically occur in older elite athletes.
- Surgical intervention is recommended to improve peak torque.
- Surgical technique is crucial to minimize complications.

BACKGROUND

Achilles tendon ruptures are devastating injuries that often occur in competitive athletes with an incidence of 18 per 100,000 person-years.[1] Regardless of treatment, the recovery for this injury is prolonged, often requiring up to 1 year of rehabilitation. In the United States, basketball is the most common cause of Achilles rupture, compared with soccer in Europe.[2,3] The injury typically occurs due to a dorsiflexion moment applied to the ankle as the gastrocnemius-soleus complex simultaneously contracts to plantar flex the ankle (eccentric load of the Achilles tendon).[4]

Achilles rupture most typically occurs in the third of fourth decade of a male athlete.[5] Recreational athletes account for 75% of all Achilles rupture, whereas competitive athletes account for 8% to 20%.[6] This injury is especially devastating for the elite athlete because of its prolonged recovery and variable outcomes. Previous literature indicates that more than 30% of professional athletes are unable to return to play following an Achilles rupture, with those who do return playing in fewer games with less playing time and performing at a lower level than their preinjury status 1 year postoperatively.[7]

Both nonoperative and operative treatments have been described for athletes with Achilles rupture. Recently, multiple randomized clinical trials have demonstrated the noninferiority of a nonoperative functional rehabilitation program for Achilles tendon rupture in the recreational athlete with regard to re-tear rates and patient-reported outcome scores.[8–12] Although differences are not found in the recreational, one must take into account the ceiling effect of patient-reported outcome scores, especially on the elite athlete. Previous studies have demonstrated differences in strength, with patients undergoing nonoperative functional rehabilitation for Achilles rupture having 10% to 18% less strength than those undergoing surgery at 18 months postoperative.[13] In the same study, there was a loss of approximately 14% in peak torque favoring the surgical group.[13] Although these differences might not be critical for most individuals, for the elite athlete it could be career ending, therefore surgical intervention is recommended for all elite athletes wishing to return to sport with Achilles ruptures.

This article reviews the management of Achilles rupture in elite athletes with the senior author's preferred surgical technique and postoperative protocol.

[a] Mayo Clinic Arizona, 5777 East Mayo Boulevard, Phoenix, AZ 85054, USA; [b] Hospital for Special Surgery, 420 East 72 Street, New York, NY 10021, USA
* Corresponding author.
E-mail address: OMalleyM@hss.edu

Orthop Clin N Am 51 (2020) 533–539
https://doi.org/10.1016/j.ocl.2020.06.009
0030-5898/20/© 2020 Elsevier Inc. All rights reserved.

Surgical Decision Making and Technique

Early evaluation and treatment for the elite athlete is crucial to minimize calf atrophy and begin the rehabilitation process. It is important to consider that many elite athletes are injured during games, and will need to travel to seek medical care. This puts them at increased risk of deep vein thrombosis (DVT). DVTs are very common in Achilles patients, with an incidence as high as 24%, increasing with increasing age.[14–16] Therefore, prophylaxis in these athletes should be highly considered, with Lovenox as the preferred method in those traveling with Achilles rupture. Clinical evaluation is typically sufficient in the diagnosis of an Achilles rupture, with a positive Thompson test indicating complete rupture. A palpable defect is typically felt at the site of rupture; however, this can be distorted acutely due to swelling. Advanced imaging or ultrasound is typically not necessary in most cases.

The current controversy regarding treatment of elite athletes is surrounding surgical technique. Investigators advocate for a minimally invasive approach or a traditional open approach. There is considerable heterogeneity in the current published literature regarding these techniques. The theoretic benefits of the minimally invasive approach is a lower wound complication rate, less scarring, and reduced operative time. The theoretic risk include an increase in sural nerve injury due to aberrant needle passage in the minimally invasive technique. A recent meta-analysis by Grassi and colleagues[17] demonstrated a decreased risk of postoperative complications for the minimally invasive technique, without a difference in the risk of re-rupture, sural nerve injury, or return to preinjury activity level. Although all studies included in this meta-analysis were randomized control trials, the patient populations were very heterogeneous, and application of these results to our elite athletes might not be wise.[17–23]

The senior author, who cares for many elite athletes, has abandoned the minimally invasive technique after using it exclusively for a year. We found that many patients had a persistent area of peri-incisional discoloration and swelling. A healthy 27-year-old patient suffered an open re-rupture at 6 months postoperatively through this area of abnormality (**Fig. 1**). We theorize that the minimally invasive technique places the large nonabsorbable suture knots in a subcutaneous position, and the reaction to the suture causes enhanced scarring and discoloration.

SURGICAL TECHNIQUE

A preoperative popliteal block is performed by anesthesia to help with the patient's postoperative analgesia. Tourniquet is applied to the affected extremity. The patient is placed in the prone position with all bony prominences well padded. It is important to ensure that the patient's feet partially come off the bed.

Bilateral lower extremities are prepped in. This is done to assess tension of the repair compared with the normal extremity. A longitudinal incision is made just medial to the Achilles tendon (see **Fig. 1**). Careful dissection is carried through the subcutaneous tissue avoiding pinching of the skin at any point. The paratenon layer is identified and a lap sponge can be used to gently clear off any adipose tissue. If any adhesions between the skin and paratenon layer are present, these are carefully dissected to ensure

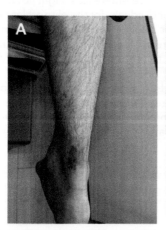
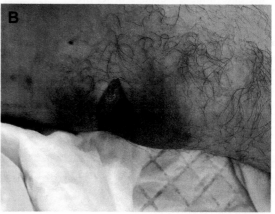

Fig. 1. Area of discoloration following minimally invasive Achilles repair (*A*), with open rupture through this area at 6 months postoperatively (*B*).

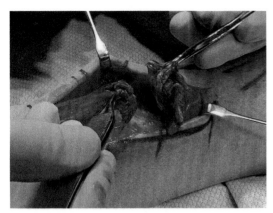

Fig. 2. Demonstration of a longitudinal incision just medial to Achilles tendon with Achilles stumps identified.

the ability to mobilize the paratenon layer for closure. An incision is created in the paratenon centered on the Achilles tendon taking care to avoid any laceration of the tendon. Dissection scissors are used to extend this paratenon incision both proximally and distally. The paratenon is carefully dissected away from the Achilles tendon both medially and laterally. This is done circumferentially for both the proximal and distal segments.

A relieving incision is made on the deep aspect of the paratenon to allow closure on the skin side. The Achilles tendon stumps are identified (Fig. 2).

Two free 2-inch Keith Needles along with 2 No. 2 nonabsorbable sutures are used for this portion of the repair. The suture is passed through the most distal portion of the Achilles tendon in the middle portion of the tendon (when assessing from anterior to posterior). This suture is then passed proximally in a modified locked Bunnell type configuration. The same is done for the proximal stump as shown in Fig. 3.

The foot is placed in maximal plantar flexion and surgeon's knots are tied on both the medial lateral aspects of the Achilles tendon and hemostatic clamp was used to hold these knots. The knees were flexed 90° in the plantar flexion resting tension was evaluated as well as inversion of the heel (Fig. 4). The operative leg was noted to have slightly more plantar flexion and inversion than the uninjured leg. Thompson's test was now negative. Final knots were then placed on both the medial and lateral limbs of the repair, and hemostatic clamps were removed. 3 to 0 Vicryl suture is used to create an epitendinous repair (see Fig. 3; Fig. 5). The wound is copiously irrigated with normal saline. The paratenon is closed using 4 to 0 Vicryl suture. The skin is closed using a combination of buried 4 to 0 Vicryl and 4 to 0 nylon suture in a horizontal mattress fashion.

The patients are placed in a splint postoperatively in 30° plantar flexion at the time of surgery. The heel and area of incision are well padded to ensure no areas of pressure injury.

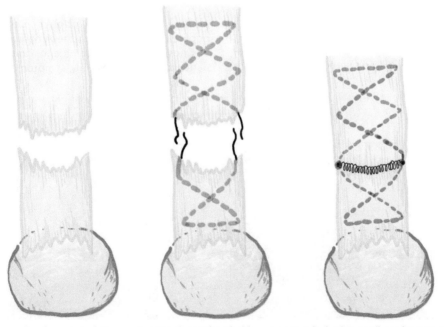

Fig. 3. Example of repair technique using No. 2 nonabsorbable suture in a locked Bunnell configuration.

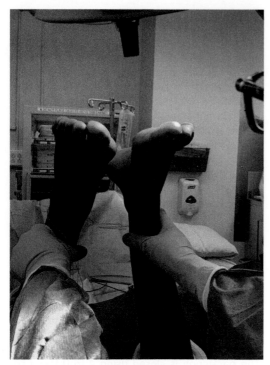

Fig. 4. Evaluation of hindfoot inversion after temporary repair using a hemostatic clamp.

POSTOPERATIVE PROTOCOL

The patients are kept in their splint for 1 week. The patient is placed on DVT prophylaxis per the surgeon's preference. Clinical check at this time is to ensure no incisional concerns. The patient is then transferred to a controlled ankle motion (CAM) boot in 30° of plantar flexion. Active plantar flexion activities are initiated at 1 week to maintain calf muscle tone and Thera-Band (Akron, OH) resistance exercises are

initiated from 15° plantar flexion to 30° plantar flexion. The patient is maintained at non–weight bearing with the use of assistive devices.

Repeat clinical examination is performed at 2 weeks postoperatively. At this time, incision is evaluated and sutures are removed. Touch down weight bearing is initiated at this time in continued 30° plantar flexion in a CAM walker boot.

At 4 weeks, the angle is reduced to 15° plantar flexion and weight bearing is progressed to 50% weight bearing. TheraBand resistance is increased; however, the range is kept from 15° plantar flexion to 30° plantar flexion. Blood flow restriction therapy is added at this time as well, in hopes of increased calf muscle girth without exposing the Achilles tendon to higher loads. Class IV laser treatment is also initiated at this time to maintain muscle health.

At 6 weeks, the patient is progressed to weight bearing as tolerated in the CAM boot in 5° of plantar flexion (1 heel lift). This is maintained until 8 weeks, at which time the patient can transition into a regular shoe. Progressive strengthening occurs thereafter, with anticipated return to sport at 6 months (**Fig. 6**).

COMPLICATIONS

As a result of the necessity for surgery in athletes hoping to return back to high-level competition, they are susceptible to the risks of surgical intervention. The most common complication for patients with Achilles rupture is deep venous thrombosis, with an incidence as high as 24%.[14,16] There is some controversy regarding treatment of thromboembolism distal to the popliteal fossa; however, the American College of Chest Physicians recommends treatment for patients who are severely symptomatic.[24] In a

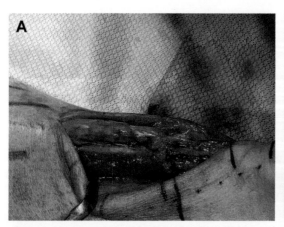
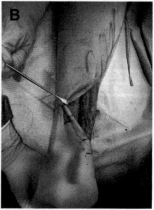

Fig. 5. (A, B) Demonstration of repair with locked Bunnell suture as well as an epitendinous repair.

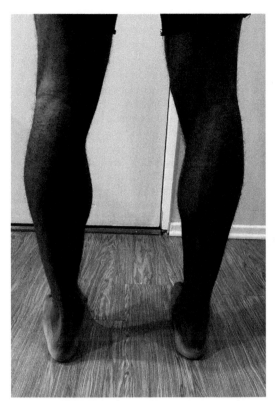

Fig. 6. Professional athlete 4 months status post open repair on the left.

recent survey study, more than 90% of practitioners treated patients with a below-knee DVT with anticoagulation, due to the fear of pulmonary embolism. Our recommended prophylaxis for patients without history of blood clot is 81 mg aspirin 2 times a day. There is basic science literature that this dosage provides the maximum antiplatelet effect of aspirin to be present for 24 hours.[25] Treatment of DVT distal to the popliteal fossa is at the surgeon's discretion.

The other common complication for repair of Achilles tendon is related to wound healing and complication. A recent meta-analysis noted increased wound issues in the open group compared with the percutaneous group; however, this difference was not present when only analyzing randomized clinical trials.[26] Recent literature indicates delayed wound healing at a rate of up to 29% with open surgery.[27] Other common complications following surgical intervention include infection, sural nerve hypoesthesia, and re-rupture.

DISCUSSION

Achilles ruptures are common injuries in our aging athletes that typically occur due to an eccentric load placed on the gastrocnemius-soleus complex. Recent literature has indicated that functional rehabilitation without surgery can lead to comparable results (patient-reported outcomes and re-rupture) to surgery, without the risk of complications.[8–12] However, it must be noted that patient-reported outcome scores do not typically capture the activities needed for our high-level competitive athletes. Consistently, surgical intervention has been noted to provide improved strength compared with functional rehabilitation. A recent meta-analysis of randomized controlled trials demonstrated improved functional outcomes by 2 different jump tests (drop counter-movement and single-leg hopping) and 1 muscular endurance test (heel-rise work) in the surgical group.[28] Peak torque has also been noted to be 10% to 14% improved in the surgical group compared with the functional rehabilitation group, as well as an improvement in strength measured by a dynamometer.[13] It is because of these differences that surgical intervention is recommended in the high-level athlete.

To help facilitate return to sport, adjuvant treatments are recommended in the postoperative setting. Lower-level laser therapy has been shown to improve muscle performance, reduce muscle fatigue, and benefit muscle repair.[29] A recent systematic review demonstrated positive effects on skeletal muscle, and the hope is that through its use, the atrophy to the gastrocnemius-soleus complex can be minimized.[30] The other modality that is used is the addition of blood flow restriction therapy (BFRT). BFRT involves placing a tourniquet on the affected extremity, allowing stimulation of muscular strength and hypertrophy at much lower loads than traditional rehabilitation. The literature is prevailing with regard to its use on Achilles rupture, limited to case reports demonstrating safe use and strength gains at this time.[31] We feel that it is a safe adjunct to traditional therapy, with a large potential upside as indicated by its use in other areas.

There is also a potential for surgical adjuvants to help promote healing of the Achilles rupture. The addition of amniotic membrane over the Achilles rupture just deep to the paratenon has been described clinically. There is a recent basic science study that demonstrated a faster healing process, reduction in the inflammatory response, and improved organization of collagen fibers in a rat model with the use of amniotic membrane.[32] At this time, amniotic membrane is not approved by the Food and Drug Administration for use on Achilles repairs;

however, no significant side effects have been noted.

The ultimate goal in treating these patients is to facilitate their return to play as quickly and safely as possible. Previous literature has demonstrated that these injuries will prevent more than 30% of professional athletes from returning to sport, and those who do typically perform at a lower level than their preinjury status.[7,33] Time to return to play is highly variable; however, previous literature on professional basketball players indicated an average of 10 months.[34]

Achilles ruptures in high-level athletes are devastating injuries that result in a loss season and a prolonged recovery. Surgery should be performed as quickly as possible, and adjuvant modalities such as low-level laser therapy and BFRT, should be used to facilitate return to sport as soon as is safe.

DISCLOSURE

The authors have nothing to disclose.

REFERENCES

1. Wertz J, Galli M, Borchers JR. Achilles tendon rupture: risk assessment for aerial and ground athletes. Sports Health 2013;5:407–9.
2. Maffulli N, Waterston SW, Squair J, et al. Changing incidence of Achilles tendon rupture in Scotland: a 15-year study. Clin J Sport Med 1999;9: 157–60.
3. Lemme NJ, Li NY, DeFroda SF, et al. Epidemiology of Achilles tendon ruptures in the United States: athletic and nonathletic injuries from 2012 to 2016. Orthop J Sports Med 2018;6. 2325967118808238.
4. Pedowitz D, Kirwan G. Achilles tendon ruptures. Curr Rev Musculoskelet Med 2013;6:285–93.
5. Maffulli N. Current concepts review - rupture of the Achilles Tendon*. J Bone Joint Surg Am 1999;81: 1019–36.
6. Leppilahti J, Orava S. Total Achilles tendon rupture. A review. Sports Med 1998;25:79–100.
7. Trofa DP, Miller JC, Jang ES, et al. ProfessionalaAthletes' return to play and performance after operative repair of an Achilles tendon rupture. Am J Sports Med 2017;45:2864–71.
8. Cetti R, Christensen SE, Ejsted R, et al. Operative versus nonoperative treatment of Achilles tendon rupture. A prospective randomized study and review of the literature. Am J Sports Med 1993;21: 791–9.
9. Ochen Y, Beks RB, van Heijl M, et al. Operative treatment versus nonoperative treatment of

Achilles tendon ruptures: systematic review and meta-analysis. BMJ 2019;364:k5120.
10. Willits K, Amendola A, Bryant D, et al. Operative versus nonoperative treatment of acute Achilles tendon ruptures: a multicenter randomized trial using accelerated functional rehabilitation. J Bone Joint Surg Am 2010;92:2767–75.
11. Wilkins R, Bisson LJ. Operative versus nonoperative management of acute Achilles tendon ruptures: a quantitative systematic review of randomized controlled trials. Am J Sports Med 2012;40(9): 2154–60. Available at: https://www.ncbi.nlm.nih. gov/pubmed/22802271.
12. Jiang N, Wang B, Chen A, et al. Operative versus nonoperative treatment for acute Achilles tendon rupture: a meta-analysis based on current evidence. Int Orthop 2012;36(4):765–73. Available at: https://www.ncbi.nlm.nih.gov/pubmed/22159659.
13. Lantto I, Heikkinen J, Flinkkila T, et al. A prospective randomized trial comparing surgical and nonsurgical treatments of acute Achilles tendon ruptures. Am J Sports Med 2016;44: 2406–14.
14. Makhdom AM, Cota A, Saran N, et al. Incidence of symptomatic deep venous thrombosis after Achilles tendon rupture. J Foot Ankle Surg 2013;52: 584–7.
15. Wu Y, Mu Y, Yin L, et al. Complications in the management of acute achilles tendon rupture: a systematic review and network meta-analysis of 2060 patients. Am J Sports Med 2019;47:2251–60.
16. Çolak İ, Gülabi D, Eceviz E, et al. Incidence of venous thromboembolism after achilles tendon surgery in patients receiving thromboprophlaxis. J Am Podiatr Med Assoc 2020;110. Article3.
17. Grassi A, Amendola A, Samuelsson K, et al. Minimally invasive versus open repair for acute achilles tendon rupture: meta-analysis showing reduced complications, with similar outcomes, after minimally invasive surgery. J Bone Joint Surg Am 2018;100:1969–81.
18. Aktas S, Kocaoglu B. Open versus minimal invasive repair with Achillon device. Foot Ankle Int 2009;30: 391–7.
19. Karabinas PK, Benetos IS, Lampropoulou-Adamidou K, et al. Percutaneous versus open repair of acute Achilles tendon ruptures. Eur J Orthop Surg Traumatol 2014;24:607–13.
20. Kołodziej L, Bohatyrewicz A, Kromuszczyńska J, et al. Efficacy and complications of open and minimally invasive surgery in acute Achilles tendon rupture: a prospective randomised clinical study– preliminary report. Int Orthop 2013;37:625–9.
21. Lim J, Dalal R, Waseem M. Percutaneous vs. open repair of the ruptured Achilles tendon–a prospective randomized controlled study. Foot Ankle Int 2001;22:559–68.

22. Majewski M, Rickert M, Steinbrück K. Achilles tendon rupture. A prospective study assessing various treatment possibilities. Orthopade 2000; 29:670–6 [in German].

23. Aviña Valencia JA, Guillén Alcalá MA. Repair of acute Achilles tendon rupture. Comparative study of two surgical techniques. Acta Ortop Mex 2009; 23:125–9 [in Spanish].

24. Kearon C, Akl EA, Comerota AJ, et al. Antithrombotic therapy for VTE disease: antithrombotic therapy and prevention of thrombosis, 9th edition: American College of Chest Physicians evidence-based clinical practice guidelines. Chest 2012;141: e419S–96S.

25. Perneby C, Wallén NH, Rooney C, et al. Dose- and time-dependent antiplatelet effects of aspirin. Thromb Haemost 2006;95:652–8.

26. Yang B, Liu Y, Kan S, et al. Outcomes and complications of percutaneous versus open repair of acute Achilles tendon rupture: A meta-analysis. Int J Surg 2017;40:178–86.

27. van Maele M, Misselyn D, Metsemakers WJ, et al. Is open acute Achilles tendon rupture repair still justified? A single center experience and critical appraisal of the literature. Injury 2018;49:1947–52.

28. Zhou K, Song L, Zhang P, et al. Surgical versus nonsurgical methods for acute achilles tendon rupture: a meta-analysis of randomized controlled trials. J Foot Ankle Surg 2018;57:1191–9.

29. Ferraresi C, Hamblin MR, Parizotto NA. Low-level laser (light) therapy (LLLT) on muscle tissue: performance, fatigue and repair benefited by the power of light. Photon Lasers Med 2012;1: 267–86.

30. Alves AN, Fernandes KPS, Deana AM, et al. Effects of low-level laser therapy on skeletal muscle repair: a systematic review. Am J Phys Med Rehabil 2014; 93:1073–85.

31. Yow BG, Tennent DJ, Dowd TC, et al. Blood flow restriction training after Achilles Tendon Rupture. J Foot Ankle Surg 2018;57:635–8.

32. Nicodemo MC, Neves LR, Aguiar JC, et al. Amniotic membrane as an option for treatment of acute Achilles tendon injury in rats. Acta Cir Bras 2017; 32:125–39.

33. Trofa DP, Noback PC, Caldwell JE, et al. Professional soccer players' return to play and performance after operative repair of Achilles Tendon Rupture. Orthop J Sports Med 2018;6. 2325967118810772.

34. Lemme NJ, Li NY, Kleiner JE, et al. Epidemiology and video analysis of achilles tendon ruptures in the National Basketball Association. Am J Sports Med 2019;47:2360–6.

Jones Fracture Management in Athletes

David J. Ruta, MD[a],*, David Parker, MD[b]

KEYWORDS

• Jones fracture • Fifth metatarsal fracture • Athletes • Intramedullary screw

KEY POINTS

• Jones fractures in both elite and recreational athletes are best treated with surgical fixation, given superior results as compared to nonoperative management.
• Intramedullary screw fixation and metatarsal plating are both reasonable options for fixation of Jones fractures in athletes. Intramedullary screw fixation is considered the standard.
• Using the largest diameter intramedullary screw to optimize canal fill has shown improved healing rates in acute and chronic fracture management.
• Autogenous bone graft should supplement revision fixation. Strong consideration should be given to biologic augmentation. Revision surgery must be accompanied by evaluation for anatomic deformity and metabolic deficiencies.
• The surgeon must be confident of clinical and radiographic healing prior to return to game play. Computed tomography may be required for confirmation in the elite athlete.

BACKGROUND

Fracture of the fifth metatarsal is the most common foot fracture,[1] and is particularly common and worrisome among athletes,[2] with potential for significant loss of game time and lingering symptoms even when properly treated.[2–6] Of several classification systems, the most widely utilized is the anatomic classification, in which the proximal portion of the fifth metatarsal is divided into 3 zones.[1,7,8] Zone I is the most proximal and includes the metatarsocuboid joint and tuberosity. Injuries in this zone are typically avulsion fractures, which have good clinical outcomes following nonoperative management.[9] Zone II is just distal to Zone I and extends to the metaphyseal-diaphyseal junction, bordered by the 4/5 intermetatarsal junction. A fracture in this area represents a true Jones fracture. Zone III includes the proximal 1.5 cm of metatarsal diaphysis. Jones fractures have been associated with high nonunion rates when treated nonoperatively, up to 70%, resulting in the current standard of fixation of these injuries in the athlete.[10,11] Anatomic studies have demonstrated a vascular watershed area supplying Zone II, contributing to the lesser healing potential.[12–14] Zone II and Zone III fractures have traditionally had similar clinical outcomes and thus are usually treated in a similar fashion.[8]

The Torg classification[15,16] describes chronicity of the fracture and influences its management (Table 1). Type I fractures are acute with a narrow fracture line and absence of intramedullary sclerosis. Type II fractures show evidence of prodromal stress or potentially a delayed union, with widening of the fracture line and some evidence of intramedullary sclerosis. Type III fractures are those with obvious nonunion and complete sclerosis of the medullary canal. Because of the high nonunion rate of Jones fractures and lengthy time to weight bearing if treated nonoperatively, it is now widely accepted that athletes benefit from

[a] Bellin Health Titletown Sports Medicine and Orthopedics, 1970 S. Ridge Road, Green Bay, WI 54304, USA; [b] University of Tennessee-Campbell Clinic Orthopaedics, 1400 S. Germantown Road, Germantown, TN 38138, USA
* Corresponding author.
E-mail address: david.j.ruta@gmail.com

Orthop Clin N Am 51 (2020) 541–553
https://doi.org/10.1016/j.ocl.2020.06.010
0030-5898/20/© 2020 Elsevier Inc. All rights reserved.

Table 1
Torg classification system for proximal fifth metatarsal fractures

Torg Classification	Radiographic Characteristics	
Type I (acute fracture)	• No intramedullary sclerosis • Fracture line with sharp margins and no widening • Minimal cortical hypertrophy • Minimal evidence of periosteal reaction	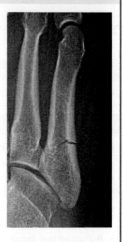
Type II (delayed union/prodromal onset)	• Fracture line involving both cortices with associated periosteal reaction • Widened fracture line with adjacent radiolucency (because of bone resorption) • Evidence of intramedullary sclerosis	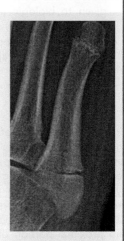
Type III (nonunion)	• Wide fracture line • Evidence of periosteal reaction and radiolucency • Complete obliteration of the medullary canal at the fracture site by sclerotic bone	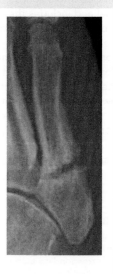

Adapted from Torg JS, Balduini FC, Zelko RR, et al. Fractures of the base of the fifth metatarsal distal to the tuberosity. Classification and guidelines for non-surgical and surgical management. J Bone Joint Surg Am 1984;66(2):209-214.

surgical fixation.[6,10] Multiple studies have demonstrated a high union rate (80%–100%) with high rate of return to sport (85%–100%) after surgical intervention.[8,17–22] Intramedullary screws are the most common surgical treatment, with some advocating for plate fixation and other alternative constructs, particularly under specific situations.[19,23–26]

EPIDEMIOLOGY

Despite the prevalence of fifth metatarsal fractures in both the athletic and general population,[2] there remains a paucity of epidemiologic studies on the subject. Seventy percent of metatarsal fractures occur at the proximal fifth metatarsal.[27] Shoe wear, a sudden increase in physical activity, certain anatomic variations, and mechanism of injury have all been reported as contributing factors to Jones fractures in all populations.[20,28,29] Acute (Torg type I) Jones fractures can occur with a high-energy abduction force on the forefoot while the ankle is plantar-flexed and inverted, but may also be caused by a rapid increase in high-level repetitive impact, as with an athlete's expedited training regimen.[30,31] In their retrospective analysis, Kane and colleagues[32] supported mechanism of injury as a predictor for fifth metatarsal fracture location. Hindfoot varus, forefoot adduction, cavus foot, and genu varum are all reported to contribute increased load to the foot's lateral column.[28,29] In a case-control study on 51 athletes, those at the greatest risk for a Jones fracture were individuals with long, straight, narrow fifth metatarsals and an adducted forefoot.[33] In older populations, women account for a greater proportion of fifth metatarsal fractures with a male predominance in younger populations. The athlete's fifth metatarsal endures tremendous strain, with some reporting that strain to be maximal at 30° to 50° of foot supination.[11]

PRESENTATION AND EVALUATION

The athlete presenting with a fifth metatarsal fracture will typically have sustained an acute injury, commonly during a pivot or landing a jump on the lateral border of his or her foot. A direct blow is less common. In some, an increasingly present prodromal pain about the lateral border of the foot will precede the acute injury by several weeks, indicating a stress component to the injury. Type I fractures may have more impressive clinical findings than Type II or III because of the acuity of the fracture.[11] Clinical evaluation of the athlete's hindfoot alignment is essential, as this will guide subsequent inserts or other orthoses. Porter and colleagues[16] showed 29% of Jones fracture patients had 2° of hindfoot valgus or less and an average calcaneal pitch of 48.8° (range, 37°–59°). These are in comparison to the typically cited normal population values of 0°-5° hindfoot valgus and 10°-30° calcaneal pitch,[34] supporting cavus as a contributing factor.

When the patient is able, a weight-bearing standard 3-view radiographic series should be performed while evaluating Jones fractures. The oblique view is commonly the most helpful for anatomic classification, although all views should be considered to most accurately assess the fracture location and pattern. Particularly if the patient is in too much pain to bear weight for radiographs, adding mild supination to the lateral view can minimize osseous overlap, allowing improved visualization of the fracture line (**Fig. 1**). Computed tomography (CT) is reserved for evaluation of delayed or nonunion or to confirm healing, particularly prior to an athlete's return to game play. CT is also helpful in diagnosing questionable repeat fracture following repeat injury with acute pain, in a previously healed fracture. MRI of the foot is more applicable when the physician has a broad differential diagnosis in mind, including a possible pending stress fracture of the fifth metatarsal.[11]

MANAGEMENT

Nonoperative management of Type II and Type III fifth metatarsal fractures remains an appropriate option in the more sedentary patient, and particularly those with greater surgical risk. It is accepted that operative management is indicated and is the standard of care for athletes.[6,10] Surgical fixation is increasingly common among nonathletes as well because of the superior union rate and enabled earlier return to daily activities and sports at any level.[7,10] Polytrauma may also be considered a relative indication for fixation, with the goal of earlier mobilization, thereby decreasing the medical and economic impact that stems from a more prolonged recovery. This is a similar concept to fixation of humeral shaft fractures in the polytrauma patient.[35,36]

Intramedullary Screw Fixation

There is debate about which fixation device is the most appropriate for Zone II and III fractures. Intramedullary screw fixation is the most common method of fixation and is accepted as the

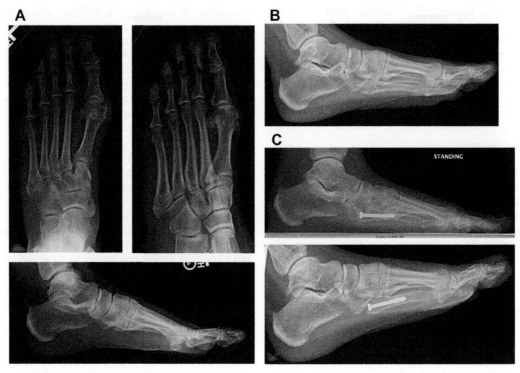

Fig. 1. (A) This injury radiographic series of a middle-aged, female recreational athlete shows the metatarsal base fracture line to be seemingly indicated for and amenable to intramedullary screw fixation. (B) The addition of a mildly supinated lateral view confirms fracture characterization. (C) Note how adding this view postoperatively can also assist with additional cortical visualization, confirming a fully healed fracture.

standard for acute, subacute, and chronic fractures (**Figs. 2** and **3**).[6,10,11,19,37] Many clinical and biomechanical studies have investigated screw specifications for further outcome optimization. These have evaluated the changes in fatigue strength with solid versus cannulated screws, with varying diameter, and with differing composition.[5,38–45] Fracture-specific screws have been developed, which are widely utilized. Partially threaded solid screws with a screw head have emerged as the most commonly studied implant, producing reliably good clinical and radiographic outcomes.[46,47] Most recently, different fracture-specific screws have undergone individual study also.[38,39,48]

There is now an increasing variety of screws for intramedullary fixation, including nearly all combinations of solid versus cannulated (sometimes finely cannulated), headed versus headless, and partially threaded versus variable pitch fully threaded. The starting point for the drill's guidewire and ultimately screw insertion has been studied, namely the traditionally recommended high and inside versus alteration of this position if strictly striving for the center of the intramedullary canal.[49] This starting point can influence iatrogenic malreduction and risk

of the screw head impinging on the cuboid, resulting in residual hardware-associated symptoms.[50] This concern has produced renewed considerations for a headless screw, a headed beveled screw, or plate fixation of the fifth metatarsal. Fully expounding each of these topics is beyond the scope of this article. In summary, literature has supported several findings:

- Solid screws have demonstrated superior fatigue strength compared with cannulated screws in biomechanical studies.[41,46]
- A clear difference in clinical outcomes between solid and cannulated screws has not been demonstrated, despite their in vitro biomechanical differences.[11,16,47]
- Authors agree that screw diameter should be maximized within the diaphyseal canal for improved thread purchase.[6,40,51]

Plate Fixation

Although intramedullary screw fixation is the standard for surgical management of Jones fractures,[6,10] concerns and limitations with that

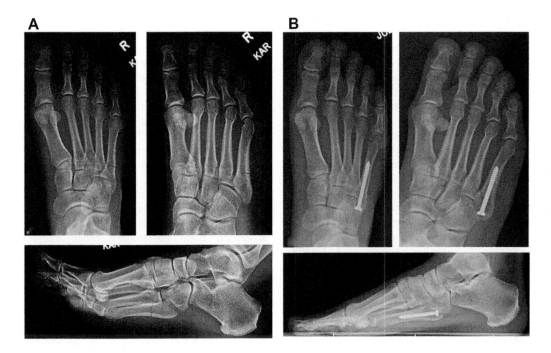

Fig. 2. (*A*) Preoperative and (*B*) postoperative radiographs showing successful management of a Zone III, Torg I Jones fracture with intramedullary fixation, utilizing a fracture-specific screw. The patient was a young, large man, active in the military. Note again the reduced metatarsal overlap in the preoperative mildly supinated lateral view.

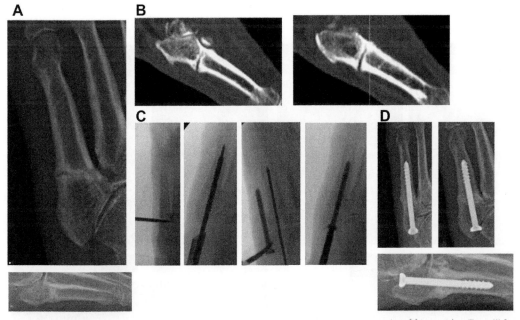

Fig. 3. (*A*) Preoperative radiographs and (*B*) CT of a recreationally athletic woman in her fifties, with a Torg III fracture. (*C*) The nonunion site was excised and prepared through an open approach, drilling, and feathering with an osteotome. The sclerotic canal was re-established with a cannulated drill, alternating between forward and reverse. This was tapped to maximize canal fill, and the tentative screw length compared alongside the bone under fluoroscopy. Calcaneal autograft was applied followed by a solid partially threaded fracture-specific screw. (*D*) By 4 months, she had returned to her baseline activity level, asymptomatic.

technique remain. Some authors have reported rates of nonunion or refracture in athletes following screw fixation between 4% and 12%, with up to a 30% refracture rate in elite athletes.[19,20,52,53] Although most reports describe time to refracture to be within 6 to 8 months, there are described refractures at 24 months postoperatively.[20,53]

Biomechanical contributions to these refractures have been investigated, with results increasing some surgeons' interest in plate fixation of Jones fractures. Placement on the tension-sided plantar surface has shown superior resistance to the tensile forces experienced by the fifth metatarsal.[44,54] Functioning as a tension band, such placement also inhibits plantar lateral gap formation, which has been shown to be the most common site of persistent cortical gap and delayed union.[55,56] Although an intramedullary screw gains stability by axial compression, the relatively softer proximal tuberosity may not always allow optimal rigid fixation at the screw head-bone interface.[6,20,57] It has also been noted that the vector of screw fixation is oriented oblique relative to the tensile forces on the metatarsal.[58] Further, a screw has been shown to impart less torsional control between the fracture fragments.[58] A combination of these findings may predispose an athlete's Jones

fracture managed with intramedullary screw fixation to potential for delayed union, nonunion, or refracture upon resuming high-level impact.

Most authors agree that a comminuted proximal fifth metatarsal fracture is an indication for plate fixation.[25,59] This is owing to the ability for multiple points of fixation, as opposed to the single axial vector produced by an intramedullary screw (**Fig. 4**). Further, as in fractures elsewhere, comminution is not a length-stable fracture pattern, and is therefore more effectively managed with a plate with locking options.[25] Proponents of plate fixation also argue that in all fracture types, the softer proximal metaphyseal fragment is more rigidly fixed with a locking plate construct.[58] Those fractures with a more dramatic bow to the metatarsal may also be more reliably stabilized with a contouring plate, as a more bowed metatarsal will be distracted at its lateral cortex if not fixed with the correct intramedullary screw length. This is produced by advancement of a straight screw within a curved bone[60] (**Fig. 5**). Depending on the fracture location, degree of metatarsal bowing, and screw length options, this can be a difficult balance to achieve.

Some surgeons report the surgical approach for plate fixation to be its own benefit, as direct fracture reduction is permitted and visual

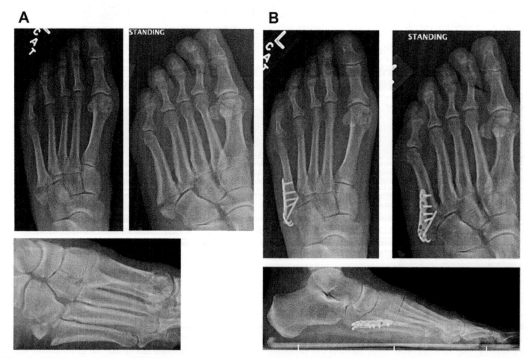

Fig. 4. (A) Preoperative and (B) 3-month postoperative radiographs showing open reduction internal fixation of a displaced, comminuted, intra-articular fifth metatarsal base fracture using plate fixation.

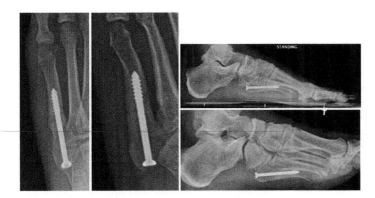

Fig. 5. Eight weeks status post intramedullary screw fixation of a Zone III Torg II fracture in a high-level collegiate lacrosse player, confirming early healing. As demonstrated on oblique and lateral views, a longer screw in this bowed metatarsal would have distracted the plantar and lateral cortices, increasing the athlete's risk of delayed or nonunion.

compression confirmed, as well as grafting and/or biologic augmentation facilitated without a separate surgical approach.[54] As the nutrient artery enters the fifth metatarsal on its dorsomedial aspect, a lateral open approach is not considered a threat to the biologic component of fracture healing.[11] Re-establishment of the medullary canal can be technically difficult and can risk cortical perforation in a Torg III fracture.[6,11] Some authors feel this step is more easily accomplished with an open plating approach, still with healing rates reported as 100% in Young and colleagues'[54] series of 38 athletes undergoing plate fixation, with 14 classified as Torg II and 4 as Torg III.

There are, however, also limitations with plate fixation. Refractures still occur, with Young and colleagues[54] reporting a 10.5% refracture rate in their retrospective series of athletic stress fractures. Unique to plate fixation is the introduction of cortical stress risers at the screw holes,[10] with 3 of the 4 refractures in this series occurring through a screw hole.[54] The extramedullary implant can be a persistent focus of irritability, particularly in an athlete wearing low-profile footwear. Even in series reporting favorable outcomes with Jones fracture plating, patients requested additional surgery for hardware removal in 24% to 31% of cases.[54,61] Plate removal following fracture healing in an elite athlete is unfortunately accompanied by a further increased concern for refracture at the residual screw holes, which would remain stress risers even if a prophylactic intramedullary screw were to be placed upon plate removal. There is also concern about how best to manage residual screw fragments if refracture following a failed plate is to be revised to an intramedullary screw.[10,50] The canal may be blocked by such screw fragments, and overdrilling for removal renders even greater stress risers and even greater potential for intraoperative fracture

upon intramedullary screw placement. With the open exposure, there is also potential for sural neuritis, with a 5% to 25% incidence reported, although these typically fully resolve within 6 weeks.[25,58] Although plate fixation is supported by the previously mentioned clinical and biomechanical data, it also presents unique hurdles. It is to the surgeon's benefit to be familiar with this technique, particularly for management of comminuted fractures.

Biologic Consideration and Augmentation

In an attempt to achieve reliable healing and expedite return to game play, there is increasing interest in biologic augmentation for Jones fractures. This is particularly important with the trend toward single-sport specialization.[62] These osteobiologics may be incorporated at the time of surgery and/or in the postoperative period. Options include direct injectables and indirect stimulation via systemic treatment. Bone marrow aspirate concentrate (BMAC), platelet-rich technologies, pulsed electromagnetic field osseous stimulation, and vitamin D supplementation are some of the more commonly employed technologies. These are most effective when also coupled with a multidisciplinary team approach to the athlete's nutritional, hormonal, and emotional well-being, with providers skilled in endocrinology, nutrition, physical therapy, and sports psychology counseling all playing important roles.[62]

Although data demonstrating definitive efficacy and commercial standardization of product consistency are currently lacking,[63] the multiple means by which BMAC may be administered make it an attractive augmentation. These include open intraoperative and percutaneous injections, the latter able to be performed in a clinic or training room. Improved healing rates have been reported with isolated use and in combination with the osteoconductive properties of demineralized bone matrix (DBM).[64] Hunt and Anderson[6] reported 100% clinical and radiographic union and return to previous level of athletic competition by an average of 12.3 weeks in 21 elite athletes undergoing surgical management of Jones refractures or nonunions. All underwent solid intramedullary screw fixation, 8 also receiving combined iliac crest BMAC and DBM. There were no clinical or radiographic differences observed between these patients and those receiving cancellous autograft.

Increased area of bone bridging and earlier healing rates are among the multiple benefits reported from a systematic review comparing long-bone fractures in animals treated with platelet-rich plasma compared with a control group.[65] Clinical studies in people have been less conclusive. The addition of pulsed electromagnetic field (PEMF) osseous stimulation to surgical fixation of fifth metatarsal delayed unions or nonunions showed decreased time to union and increased production of bone morphogenic proteins in a randomized controlled study of 8 fractures.[66]

Vitamin D [25(OH)D$_3$] levels less than 30 ng/mL in soccer players have been shown to be associated with a significantly increased risk for fifth metatarsal stress fracture. The risk of fracture was nearly 3 times in those with serum levels less than 20 ng/mL.[67,68] The risk of hypovitaminosis D is especially high during winter and spring training and north of 40° latitude.[69] Multiple studies have shown an association between hypovitaminosis D and lower extremity stress fractures in military recruits[70–72] as well as within the general orthopedic trauma population.[73,74] Some authors suggest that athletes with demonstrated 25(OH)D$_3$ deficiency or those at high risk based upon training season and/or geography should undergo aggressive supplementation, with a goal of 50 ng/mL,[62,75] although there is not high-level evidence to demonstrate a preventive effect of vitamin D maintenance against stress fractures. Work-up for nonunion should include vitamin D and thyroid hormone levels.[76]

COMPLICATIONS

Despite the largely successful outcomes following surgical management of Jones fracture, there are known complications. Nonunion or refracture has been reported in up to 12% of patients following intramedullary screw fixation (30% refracture rate in elite athletes)[19,20,52,53] and 10.5% following plate fixation.[54] Refractures and nonunions can be associated with insufficient fixation, too aggressive of a postoperative rehabilitation, deformity (including subtle), and biologic insufficiency at the fracture site.[6] Clinical and radiographic evaluation of nonunions and refractures should be similar to that described earlier for acute fractures. In addition to surgery at the fracture site, realignment including calcaneal and/or first metatarsal osteotomy is indicated for failed Jones fracture management in the context of subtle cavus.[77,78]

A recurrent Jones fracture that is nondisplaced, with an intact and appropriately sized implant, and without contributing deformity may initially undergo an attempt at nonoperative management with cast or boot immobilization, nonweight bearing, and commonly use of a bone stimulator.[10] Percutaneous administration of BMAC/DBM or autograft may be used as augmentation.[6] In these circumstances, careful consideration should still be given to the reason for refracture, with realignment osteotomies as indicated and metabolic evaluation performed.

Revision Surgery

If it is determined that the original implant in a refracture was undersized or has mechanically failed, revision surgery is indicated. In a retrospective analysis of 55 athletes with Zone II fractures, 4 (7.3%) patients refractured at a mean 8 months after surgery. All were competitive athletes who had received small-diameter solid or cannulated screw fixation. Three went on to union following revision surgery with a larger-diameter solid screw, prompting authors to recommend maximizing screw diameter within the canal.[79] Hunt and Anderson[6] found refractures after index intramedullary screw fixation to occur at a mean of 32.8 weeks (8.2 months) postoperatively. In their review of 21 elite athletes undergoing revision surgery for fracture or nonunion, 17 received a larger screw diameter upon revision. These were augmented with autograft or a combination of BMAC and DBM. All patients demonstrated clinical and radiographic healing, returning to their previous level of competition at an average of 12.3 weeks. This further supports the recommendation for maximizing canal fill. Bernstein and colleagues[58] employed plantar plating with autograft to treat 4 acute Jones fractures and 4 refractures in elite athletes. All patients achieved clinical and radiographic union at an average 6.5 weeks, with impact allowed at 12.3 weeks. All returned to their previous level of competition.[58] Authors agree that when managing established nonunions (Torg III), it is important to ream and reconstitute the medullary canal, while carefully avoiding perforation. In addition, nonunion fixation is typically augmented with autograft or other biologic means.[6,58] Return to play prior to full union is a risk factor for delayed/nonunion and refracture,[31] prompting elite athletes to commonly undergo CT scan prior to unrestricted impact, particularly following revision fixation.[10,11]

Symptomatic Hardware

Even with successful union, symptomatic hardware can present the athlete with nagging, distracting symptoms, limiting performance intensity. This is reported in up to 30% of patients following intramedullary screw fixation with a traditional screw[18,80,81] and up to 31% following plate fixation.[54,61] With the advent of the fracture-specific screw, irritation at the screw head has become rarely reported.[11] Symptomatic hardware can be managed with shoe modifications, hardware removal, or hardware exchange.[80] Hardware removal from the fifth metatarsal base in the active athlete should not be undertaken without careful consideration, as the residual screw hole(s) will remain a stress riser.[10] It is recommended that fifth metatarsal fixation remain in place throughout the duration

of an athlete's career, to decrease the risk of refracture upon removal.[82]

As described earlier, the holes from a plate's cortical screws have been shown to be a common site of refracture.[10,54] These remain even if a hardware exchange is performed, with a prophylactic intramedullary screw placed. A symptomatic intramedullary screw head can occur from impingement on the cuboid, which may be secondary to a slightly proud implant or the originally determined starting point[11,49,50] (Fig. 6). There are differing opinions regarding how this complication is best managed. Some authors indicate that prevention is key, using a headless screw as the index implant if anatomy is such that impingement on the cuboid is likely[54] or performing a cuboid osteoplasty to access the ideal starting point.[49] Others suggest implant exchange to a headless screw only if a symptomatic screw head develops.[1] Still others advocate performing an implant exchange to another headed screw, although with intentional recess of the head further into the metatarsal base.[11] There is not a consensus within the literature for any 1 solution. A headed fracture-specific screw with a focal bevel within the head has been developed, to allow this low-profile edge to face the cuboid. At the time of this writing, there are no published outcomes on this implant modification.

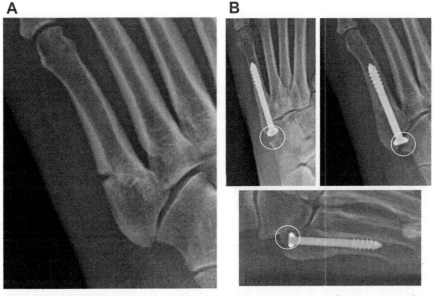

Fig. 6. (*A*) Preoperative and (*B*) postoperative radiographs demonstrating successful open autografting and intramedullary fixation of a Torg III fracture. Despite resolution of preoperative symptoms, a mild ongoing ache and tenderness were present overlying the screw head. Note the cuboid scalloping present on all 3 postoperative views, consistent with impingement from the adjacent screw head. The patient ultimately elected for screw removal, declining implant exchange.

SUMMARY

Today, literature supports the standard of care for Jones fracture management in the athlete to be surgical fixation. Fracture-specific intramedullary screws, which are partially threaded and solid, are the most commonly utilized implant. Multiple studies have highlighted the importance of maximizing canal fill. At the same time, careful attention must also be given to avoiding an overly long screw and optimizing starting point, while also attempting to avoid impingement on the cuboid. There is sound biomechanical and clinical support for plate fixation, shown effective in simple acute management and revision surgery, although this may be most appropriately employed for comminuted fractures. The surgeon should give consideration to the unique hurdles that may come with plate failure and revision thereof.

Multiple studies have consistently supported good-to-excellent outcomes with surgical treatment of Jones fractures. Additional research on metabolic risks, mechanical contribution, and optimization of postoperative protocols will allow further improvement to management. Evaluation of the athlete's alignment and metabolic profile should be part of standard Jones fracture treatment, although this warrants particularly careful consideration in the management of nonunion or refracture. Intramedullary screw fixation with bone grafting, maximized canal fill, and biologic augmentation, frequently with external bone stimulation, is the mainstay of revision surgery. Ongoing study into risk factor mitigation and implant optimization will facilitate increasingly improved outcomes and aid in surgical decision making for this common athletic foot injury.

CLINICS CARE POINTS

Literature supports increased union rate and decreased time to impact and return to play with operative management of Jones fractures (both Zone 2 and 3 base of fifth metatarsal fractures). Athletes presenting with this injury should be counseled in this and offered surgery.

Evaluation should include query of prodromal pain, examination of lower extremity mechanical axis, and analysis of metabolic profile, particularly vitamin D level if located in northern latitudes and/or during winter/spring training. Open nonunion takedown with autologous bone grafting or a combination of concentrated bone marrow aspirate and demineralized bone

matrix with internal fixation is supported as appropriate management for symptomatic Jones fracture nonunions (Torg III).

One must take care to safely maximize screw diameter during revision surgery for refracture. Patients should be counseled in the risk of symptomatic hardware with either intramedullary screw or plate fixation, although with a greater incidence of such and potential need for hardware removal following plate fixation.

DISCLOSURE

Neither author has any relevant disclosures.

REFERENCES

1. Japjec M, Starešinić M, Starjački M, et al. Treatment of proximal fifth metatarsal bone fractures in athletes. Injury 2015;46(Suppl 6):S134–6.
2. Kaplan LD, Jost PW, Honkamp N, et al. Incidence and variance of foot and ankle injuries in elite college football players. Am J Orthop (Belle Mead NJ) 2011;40(1):40–4.
3. Bigsby E, Halliday R, Middleton RG, et al. Functional outcome of fifth metatarsal fractures. Injury 2014;45(12):2009–12.
4. Carreira DS, Sandilands SM. Radiographic factors and effect of fifth metatarsal Jones and diaphyseal stress fractures on participation in the NFL. Foot Ankle Int 2013;34(4):518–22.
5. Porter DA, Rund AM, Dobslaw R, et al. Comparison of 4.5- and 5.5-mm cannulated stainless steel screws for fifth metatarsal Jones fracture fixation. Foot Ankle Int 2009;30(1):27–33.
6. Hunt KJ, Anderson RB. Treatment of Jones fracture nonunions and refractures in the elite athlete: outcomes of intramedullary screw fixation with bone grafting. Am J Sports Med 2011;39(9):1948–54.
7. Quill GE. Fractures of the proximal fifth metatarsal. Orthop Clin North Am 1995;26(2):353–61.
8. Chuckpaiwong B, Queen RM, Easley ME, et al. Distinguishing Jones and proximal diaphyseal fractures of the fifth metatarsal. Clin Orthop Relat Res 2008;466(8):1966–70.
9. Akimau PI, Cawthron KL, Dakin WM, et al. Symptomatic treatment or cast immobilisation for avulsion fractures of the base of the fifth metatarsal: a prospective, randomised, single-blinded non-inferiority controlled trial. Bone Joint J 2016;98-B(6):806–11.
10. Lareau CR, Anderson RB. Jones fractures: pathophysiology and treatment. JBJS Rev 2015;3(7).
11. Porter DA. Fifth metatarsal jones fractures in the athlete. Foot Ankle Int 2018;39(2):250–8.
12. Nunley JA. Fractures of the base of the fifth metatarsal: the Jones fracture. Orthop Clin North Am 2001;32(1):171–80.

13. Shereff MJ, Yang QM, Kummer FJ, et al. Vascular anatomy of the fifth metatarsal. Foot Ankle 1991; 11(6):350–3.

14. Smith JW, Arnoczky SP, Hersh A. The intraosseous blood supply of the fifth metatarsal: implications for proximal fracture healing. Foot Ankle 1992; 13(3):143–52.

15. Torg JS, Balduini FC, Zelko RR, et al. Fractures of the base of the fifth metatarsal distal to the tuberosity. Classification and guidelines for non-surgical and surgical management. J Bone Joint Surg Am 1984;66(2):209–14.

16. Porter DA, Duncan M, Meyer SJ. Fifth metatarsal Jones fracture fixation with a 4.5-mm cannulated stainless steel screw in the competitive and recreational athlete: a clinical and radiographic evaluation. Am J Sports Med 2005;33(5):726–33.

17. Clapper MF, O'Brien TJ, Lyons PM. Fractures of the fifth metatarsal. Analysis of a fracture registry. Clin Orthop Relat Res 1995;(315):238–41.

18. Mologne TS, Lundeen JM, Clapper MF, et al. Early screw fixation versus casting in the treatment of acute Jones fractures. Am J Sports Med 2005; 33(7):970–5.

19. Murawski CD, Kennedy JG. Percutaneous internal fixation of proximal fifth metatarsal jones fractures (Zones II and III) with Charlotte Carolina screw and bone marrow aspirate concentrate: an outcome study in athletes. Am J Sports Med 2011;39(6):1295–301.

20. O'Malley M, DeSandis B, Allen A, et al. Operative treatment of fifth metatarsal jones fractures (zones II and III) in the NBA. Foot Ankle Int 2016;37(5):488–500.

21. Polzer H, Polzer S, Mutschler W, et al. Acute fractures to the proximal fifth metatarsal bone: development of classification and treatment recommendations based on the current evidence. Injury 2012;43(10):1626–32.

22. Begly JP, Guss M, Ramme AJ, et al. Return to play and performance after jones fracture in National Basketball Association Athletes. Sports Health 2016;8(4):342–6.

23. Kelly IP, Glisson RR, Fink C, et al. Intramedullary screw fixation of Jones fractures. Foot Ankle Int 2001;22(7):585–9.

24. Huh J, Glisson RR, Matsumoto T, et al. Biomechanical comparison of intramedullary screw versus low-profile plate fixation of a Jones fracture. Foot Ankle Int 2016;37(4):411–8.

25. Lee SK, Park JS, Choy WS. Locking compression plate distal ulna hook plate as alternative fixation for fifth metatarsal base fracture. J Foot Ankle Surg 2014;53(5):522–8.

26. Tomic S, Vucic V, Dobric M, et al. Treatment of acute Jones fracture with Ilizarov external minifixator: case series of six elite athletes. J Foot Ankle Surg 2013;52(3):374–9.

27. Petrisor BA, Ekrol I, Court-Brown C. The epidemiology of metatarsal fractures. Foot Ankle Int 2006; 27(3):172–4.

28. Raikin SM, Slenker N, Ratigan B. The association of a varus hindfoot and fracture of the fifth metatarsal metaphyseal-diaphyseal junction: the Jones fracture. Am J Sports Med 2008;36(7):1367–72.

29. Fleischer AE, Stack R, Klein EE, et al. Forefoot adduction is a risk factor for jones fracture. J Foot Ankle Surg 2017;56(5):917–21.

30. Jones RI. Fracture of the base of the fifth metatarsal bone by indirect violence. Ann Surg 1902;35(6): 697–700.

31. Wright RW, Fischer DA, Shively RA, et al. Refracture of proximal fifth metatarsal (Jones) fracture after intramedullary screw fixation in athletes. Am J Sports Med 2000;28(5):732–6.

32. Kane JM, Sandrowski K, Saffel H, et al. The epidemiology of fifth metatarsal fracture. Foot Ankle Spec 2015;8(5):354–9.

33. Karnovsky SC, Rosenbaum AJ, DeSandis B, et al. Radiographic analysis of National Football League players' fifth metatarsal morphology relationship to proximal fifth metatarsal fracture risk. Foot Ankle Int 2019;40(3):318–22.

34. Irwin TA, Anderson RB, Davis WH. Principles of the physical examination of the foot and ankle. In: Coughlin M, editor. Mann's surgery of the foot and ankle. 9th edition. Mosby; 2013. p. 37–60.

35. Carroll EA, Schweppe M, Langfitt M, et al. Management of humeral shaft fractures. J Am Acad Orthop Surg 2012;20(7):423–33.

36. Kubiak EN, Beebe MJ, North K, et al. Early weight bearing after lower extremity fractures in adults. J Am Acad Orthop Surg 2013;21(12):727–38.

37. Bucknam RB, Scanaliato JP, Kusnezov NA, et al. Return to weightbearing and high-impact activities following jones fracture intramedullary screw fixation. Foot Ankle Int 2020;41(4):379–86.

38. Jastifer J, McCullough KA. Fatigue bending strength of jones fracture specific screw fixation. Foot Ankle Int 2018;39(4):493–9.

39. Metzl J, Olson K, Davis WH, et al. A clinical and radiographic comparison of two hardware systems used to treat jones fracture of the fifth metatarsal. Foot Ankle Int 2013;34(7):956–61.

40. Larson CM, Almekinders LC, Taft TN, et al. Intramedullary screw fixation of Jones fractures. Analysis of failure. Am J Sports Med 2002;30(1):55–60.

41. Reese K, Litsky A, Kaeding C, et al. Cannulated screw fixation of Jones fractures: a clinical and biomechanical study. Am J Sports Med 2004; 32(7):1736–42.

42. Sides SD, Fetter NL, Glisson R, et al. Bending stiffness and pull-out strength of tapered, variable pitch screws, and 6.5-mm cancellous screws in acute Jones fractures. Foot Ankle Int 2006;27(10):821–5.

43. Orr JD, Glisson RR, Nunley JA. Jones fracture fixation: a biomechanical comparison of partially threaded screws versus tapered variable pitch screws. Am J Sports Med 2012;40(3):691–8.

44. Duplantier NL, Mitchell RJ, Zambrano S, et al. A biomechanical comparison of fifth metatarsal jones fracture fixation methods. Am J Sports Med 2018;46(5):1220–7.

45. DeVries JG, Cuttica DJ, Hyer CF. Cannulated screw fixation of Jones fifth metatarsal fractures: a comparison of titanium and stainless steel screw fixation. J Foot Ankle Surg 2011;50(2):207–12.

46. Nunley JA, Glisson RR. A new option for intramedullary fixation of Jones fractures: the Charlotte Carolina Jones Fracture System. Foot Ankle Int 2008;29(12):1216–21.

47. Nagao M, Saita Y, Kameda S, et al. Headless compression screw fixation of jones fractures: an outcomes study in Japanese athletes. Am J Sports Med 2012;40(11):2578–82.

48. Willegger M, Benca E, Hirtler L, et al. Evaluation of two types of intramedullary jones fracture fixation in a cyclic and ultimate load model. J Orthop Res 2020;38(4):911–7.

49. Watson GI, Karnovsky SC, Konin G, et al. Optimal starting point for fifth metatarsal zone II fractures: a cadaveric study. Foot Ankle Int 2017;38(7):802–7.

50. Roberts L, Bernasconi A, Netto CC, et al. Cuboid edema syndrome following fixation of proximal fifth metatarsal fractures in professional athletes. Foot Ankle Spec 2019;12(4):373–9.

51. Ochenjele G, Ho B, Switaj PJ, et al. Radiographic study of the fifth metatarsal for optimal intramedullary screw fixation of Jones fracture. Foot Ankle Int 2015;36(3):293–301.

52. Roche AJ, Calder JD. Treatment and return to sport following a Jones fracture of the fifth metatarsal: a systematic review. Knee Surg Sports Traumatol Arthrosc 2013;21(6):1307–15.

53. Lareau CR, Hsu AR, Anderson RB. Return to play in National Football League players after operative Jones fracture treatment. Foot Ankle Int 2016; 37(1):8–16.

54. Young KW, Kim JS, Lee HS, et al. Operative results of plantar plating for fifth metatarsal stress fracture. Foot Ankle Int 2020;41(4):419–27.

55. Renner C, Whyte J, Singh S, et al. Treatment of fractures of the fifth metatarsal with the XS-nail retrospective study and comparison with tension-band wiring. Arch Orthop Trauma Surg 2010; 130(9):1149–56.

56. Sarimo J, Rantanen J, Orava S, et al. Tension-band wiring for fractures of the fifth metatarsal located in the junction of the proximal metaphysis and diaphysis. Am J Sports Med 2006;34(3):476–80.

57. Glasgow MT, Naranja RJ, Glasgow SG, et al. Analysis of failed surgical management of fractures of the base

of the fifth metatarsal distal to the tuberosity: the Jones fracture. Foot Ankle Int 1996;17(8):449–57.

58. Bernstein DT, Mitchell RJ, McCulloch PC, et al. Treatment of proximal fifth metatarsal fractures and refractures with plantar plating in elite athletes. Foot Ankle Int 2018;39(12):1410–5.

59. Seyidova N, Hirtler L, Windhager R, et al. Peroneus brevis tendon in proximal 5th metatarsal fractures: anatomical considerations for safe hook plate placement. Injury 2018;49(3):720–5.

60. Horst F, Gilbert BJ, Glisson RR, et al. Torque resistance after fixation of Jones fractures with intramedullary screws. Foot Ankle Int 2004;25(12):914–9.

61. Kadar A, Ankory R, Karpf R, et al. Plate fixation of proximal fifth metatarsal fracture. J Am Podiatr Med Assoc 2015;105(5):389–94.

62. Miller TL, Kaeding CC, Rodeo SA. Emerging options for biologic enhancement of stress fracture healing in athletes. J Am Acad Orthop Surg 2020;28(1):1–9.

63. Imam MA, Holton J, Ernstbrunner L, et al. A systematic review of the clinical applications and complications of bone marrow aspirate concentrate in management of bone defects and nonunions. Int Orthop 2017;41(11):2213–20.

64. Tiedeman JJ, Connolly JF, Strates BS, et al. Treatment of nonunion by percutaneous injection of bone marrow and demineralized bone matrix. An experimental study in dogs. Clin Orthop Relat Res 1991;268:294–302.

65. Gianakos A, Zambrana L, Savage-Elliott I, et al. Platelet-rich plasma in the animal long-bone model: an analysis of basic science evidence. Orthopedics 2015;38(12):e1079–90.

66. Streit A, Watson BC, Granata JD, et al. Effect on clinical outcome and growth factor synthesis with adjunctive use of pulsed electromagnetic fields for fifth metatarsal nonunion fracture: a double-blind randomized study. Foot Ankle Int 2016;37(9): 919–23.

67. Shimasaki Y, Nagao M, Miyamori T, et al. Evaluating the risk of a fifth metatarsal stress fracture by measuring the serum 25-hydroxyvitamin D levels. Foot Ankle Int 2016;37(3):307–11.

68. Davey T, Lanham-New SA, Shaw AM, et al. Low serum 25-hydroxyvitamin D is associated with increased risk of stress fracture during Royal Marine recruit training. Osteoporos Int 2016;27(1):171–9.

69. Webb AR, Kline L, Holick MF. Influence of season and latitude on the cutaneous synthesis of vitamin D3: exposure to winter sunlight in Boston and Edmonton will not promote vitamin D3 synthesis in human skin. J Clin Endocrinol Metab 1988; 67(2):373–8.

70. Dao D, Sodhi S, Tabasinejad R, et al. Serum 25-hydroxyvitamin D levels and stress fractures in military personnel: a systematic review and meta-analysis. Am J Sports Med 2015;43(8):2064–72.

71. Lappe J, Cullen D, Haynatzki G, et al. Calcium and vitamin d supplementation decreases incidence of stress fractures in female navy recruits. J Bone Miner Res 2008;23(5):741–9.

72. McCabe MP, Smyth MP, Richardson DR. Current concept review: vitamin D and stress fractures. Foot Ankle Int 2012;33(6):526–33.

73. Andres BA, Childs BR, Vallier HA. Treatment of hypovitaminosis D in an orthopaedic trauma population. J Orthop Trauma 2018;32(4):e129–33.

74. Haines N, Kempton LB, Seymour RB, et al. The effect of a single early high-dose vitamin D supplement on fracture union in patients with hypovitaminosis D: a prospective randomised trial. Bone Joint J 2017;99-B(11):1520–5.

75. Miller JR, Dunn KW, Ciliberti LJ, et al. Association of vitamin D with stress fractures: a retrospective cohort study. J Foot Ankle Surg 2016;55(1):117–20.

76. Taylor PN, Razvi S, Pearce SH, et al. Clinical review: A review of the clinical consequences of variation in thyroid function within the reference range. J Clin Endocrinol Metab 2013;98(9):3562–71.

77. Solan M, Davies M. Nonunion of fifth metatarsal fractures. Foot Ankle Clin 2014;19(3):499–519.

78. Weinfeld SB, Haddad SL, Myerson MS. Metatarsal stress fractures. Clin Sports Med 1997;16(2):319–38.

79. Granata JD, Berlet GC, Philbin TM, et al. Failed surgical management of acute proximal fifth metatarsal (Jones) fractures: a retrospective case series and literature review. Foot Ankle Spec 2015;8(6):454–9.

80. DeLee JC, Evans JP, Julian J. Stress fracture of the fifth metatarsal. Am J Sports Med 1983;11(5):349–53.

81. Portland G, Kelikian A, Kodros S. Acute surgical management of Jones' fractures. Foot Ankle Int 2003;24(11):829–33.

82. Josefsson PO, Karlsson M, Redlund-Johnell I, et al. Jones fracture. Surgical versus nonsurgical treatment. Clin Orthop Relat Res 1994;299:252–5.

UNITED STATES POSTAL SERVICE ®

Statement of Ownership, Management, and Circulation (All Periodicals Publications Except Requester Publications)

1. Publication Title	2. Publication Number		3. Filing Date
ORTHOPEDIC CLINICS OF NORTH AMERICA	950 – 920		9/18/2020

4. Issue Frequency	5. Number of Issues Published Annually	6. Annual Subscription Price
JAN, APR, JUL, OCT	4	$344.00

7. Complete Mailing Address of Known Office of Publication (Not printer) (Street, city, county, state, and ZIP+4®)

ELSEVIER INC.
230 Park Avenue, Suite 800
New York, NY 10169

Contact Person
Malathi Samayan
Telephone: (Include area code)
91-44-4299-4507

8. Complete Mailing Address of Headquarters or General Business Office of Publisher (Not printer)

ELSEVIER INC.
230 Park Avenue, Suite 800
New York, NY 10169

9. Full Names and Complete Mailing Addresses of Publisher, Editor, and Managing Editor (Do not leave blank)

Publisher (Name and complete mailing address)

DOLORES MELON, ELSEVIER INC.
1600 JOHN F KENNEDY BLVD. SUITE 1800
PHILADELPHIA, PA 19103-2899

Editor (Name and complete mailing address)

LAUREN BOYLE, ELSEVIER INC.
1600 JOHN F KENNEDY BLVD. SUITE 1800
PHILADELPHIA, PA 19103-2899

Managing Editor (Name and complete mailing address)

PATRICK MANLEY, ELSEVIER INC.
1600 JOHN F KENNEDY BLVD. SUITE 1800
PHILADELPHIA, PA 19103-2899

10. Owner (Do not leave blank. If the publication is owned by a corporation, give the name and address of the corporation immediately followed by the names and addresses of all stockholders owning or holding 1 percent or more of the total amount of stock. If not owned by a corporation, give the names and addresses of the individual owners. If owned by a partnership or other unincorporated firm, give its name and address as well as those of each individual owner. If the publication is published by a nonprofit organization, give its name and address.)

Full Name	Complete Mailing Address
WHOLLY OWNED SUBSIDIARY OF REED/ELSEVIER, US HOLDINGS	1600 JOHN F KENNEDY BLVD. SUITE 1800 PHILADELPHIA, PA 19103-2899

11. Known Bondholders, Mortgagees, and Other Security Holders Owning or Holding 1 Percent or More of Total Amount of Bonds, Mortgages, or Other Securities. If none, check box. ▶ ☐ None

Full Name	Complete Mailing Address
N/A	

12. Tax Status (For completion by nonprofit organizations authorized to mail at nonprofit rates) (Check one)
The purpose, function, and nonprofit status of this organization and the exempt status for federal income tax purposes:
☒ Has Not Changed During Preceding 12 Months
☐ Has Changed During Preceding 12 Months (Publisher must submit explanation of change with this statement)

PS Form 3526, July 2014 (Page 1 of 4 (see instructions page 4)) PSN: 7530-01-000-9931   PRIVACY NOTICE: See our privacy policy on www.usps.com

13. Publication Title	14. Issue Date for Circulation Data Below
ORTHOPEDIC CLINICS OF NORTH AMERICA	JULY 2020

15. Extent and Nature of Circulation			Average No. Copies Each Issue During Preceding 12 Months	No. Copies of Single Issue Published Nearest to Filing Date
a. Total Number of Copies (Net press run)			201	175
b. Paid Circulation (By Mail and Outside the Mail)	(1)	Mailed Outside-County Paid Subscriptions Stated on PS Form 3541 (Include paid distribution above nominal rate, advertiser's proof copies, and exchange copies)	64	53
	(2)	Mailed In-County Paid Subscriptions Stated on PS Form 3541 (Include paid distribution above nominal rate, advertiser's proof copies, and exchange copies)	0	0
	(3)	Paid Distribution Outside the Mails Including Sales Through Dealers and Carriers, Street Vendors, Counter Sales, and Other Paid Distribution Outside USPS®	98	93
	(4)	Paid Distribution by Other Classes of Mail Through the USPS (e.g. First-Class Mail®)	0	0
c. Total Paid Distribution (Sum of 15b (1), (2), (3), and (4))		▶	162	146
d. Free or Nominal Rate Distribution (By Mail and Outside the Mail)	(1)	Free or Nominal Rate Outside-County Copies included on PS Form 3541	22	16
	(2)	Free or Nominal Rate In-County Copies Included on PS Form 3541	0	0
	(3)	Free or Nominal Rate Copies Mailed at Other Classes Through the USPS (e.g. First-Class Mail)	0	0
	(4)	Free or Nominal Rate Distribution Outside the Mail (Carriers or other means)	0	0
e. Total Free or Nominal Rate Distribution (Sum of 15d (1), (2), (3) and (4))		▶	22	16
f. Total Distribution (Sum of 15c and 15e)		▶	184	162
g. Copies not Distributed (See Instructions to Publishers #4 (page #3))		▶	17	13
h. Total (Sum of 15f and g)		▶	201	175
i. Percent Paid (15c divided by 15f times 100)			88.04%	90.12%

* If you are claiming electronic copies, go to line 16 on page 3. If you are not claiming electronic copies, skip to line 17 on page 3.

16. Electronic Copy Circulation	Average No. Copies Each Issue During Preceding 12 Months	No. Copies of Single Issue Published Nearest to Filing Date
a. Paid Electronic Copies ▶		
b. Total Paid Print Copies (Line 15c) + Paid Electronic Copies (Line 16a) ▶		
c. Total Print Distribution (Line 15f) + Paid Electronic Copies (Line 16a) ▶		
d. Percent Paid (Both Print & Electronic Copies) (16b divided by 16c × 100) ▶		

☒ I certify that 50% of all my distributed copies (electronic and print) are paid above a nominal price.

17. Publication of Statement of Ownership

☒ If the publication is a general publication, publication of this statement is required. Will be printed in the OCTOBER 2020 issue of this publication. ☐ Publication not required.

18. Signature and Title of Editor, Publisher, Business Manager, or Owner	Date
Malathi Samayan - Distribution Controller *Malathi Samayan*	9/18/2020

I certify that all information furnished on this form is true and complete. I understand that anyone who furnishes false or misleading information on this form or who omits material or information requested on the form may be subject to criminal sanctions (including fines and imprisonment) and/or civil sanctions (including civil penalties).

PS Form 3526, July 2014 (Page 2 of 4)   PRIVACY NOTICE: See our privacy policy on www.usps.com

Moving?

Make sure your subscription moves with you!

To notify us of your new address, find your **Clinics Account Number** (located on your mailing label above your name), and contact customer service at:

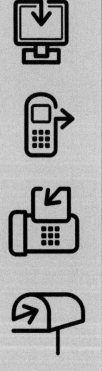

Email: journalscustomerservice-usa@elsevier.com

800-654-2452 (subscribers in the U.S. & Canada)
314-447-8871 (subscribers outside of the U.S. & Canada)

Fax number: 314-447-8029

Elsevier Health Sciences Division
Subscription Customer Service
3251 Riverport Lane
Maryland Heights, MO 63043

*To ensure uninterrupted delivery of your subscription, please notify us at least 4 weeks in advance of move.

Printed and bound by CPI Group (UK) Ltd, Croydon, CR0 4YY

08/05/2025

01864697-0016